AF441705

# ULTRASONICALLY GUIDED PUNCTURE TECHNIQUE

edited by
Hans Henrik Holm and Jørgen Kvist Kristensen

MUNKSGAARD

Ultrasonically Guided Puncture Technique
1st edition, 1st impression

Copyright © 1980 Munksgaard, Copenhagen

Cover by Finn Andersen

No part of this publication may be reproduced, stored in a retrieval system or
transmitted in any form or in a retrieval system or transmitted in any form or by
any means, electronic, mechanical, photocopying, recording or otherwise without
prior permission by the copyright owner.

Printed in Denmark by Villadsen & Christensen, Copenhagen

ISBN 87-16-8459-4

# List of Contributors

**Orla Als, M. D.**
Ultrasound Laboratory
Herlev Hospital, University of Copenhagen
2730 Herlev, Copenhagen
Denmark

**Jens Bang, M. D.**
Director of Ultrasound Laboratory
Department of Gynecology and Obstetrics Y
Rigshospitalet, University of Copenhagen
Blegdamsvej 9
2100 Copenhagen
Denmark

**Flemming Burcharth, M. D.**
Department of Surgical Gastroenterology D
Herlev Hospital, University of Copenhagen
2730 Herlev, Copenhagen
Denmark

**Jens Gammelgaard, M. D.**
Ultrasound Laboratory
Herlev Hospital, University of Copenhagen
2730 Herlev, Copenhagen
Denmark

**Søren Hancke, M. D.**
Ultrasound Laboratory
Herlev Hospital, University of Copenhagen
2730 Herlev, Copenhagen
Denmark

**Ole Boll Henriksen, M. D.**
Department of Pathological Anatomy
Herlev Hospital, University of Copenhagen
2730 Herlev, Copenhagen
Denmark

**Hans-Erik Hjelmroth, Research Engineer**
Institute of Biomedical Engineering
Park Allé 345
2600 Glostrup, Copenhagen
Denmark

**Hans Henrik Holm, M. D., Ph. D.**
Director of Ultrasound Laboratory
Chief Surgeon, Department of Urology H
Herlev Hospital, University of Copenhagen
2730 Herlev, Copenhagen
Denmark

**Grete Krag Jacobsen, M. D.**
Department of Pathological Anatomy
Herlev Hospital, University of Copenhagen
2730 Herlev, Copenhagen
Denmark

**Flemming Jensen, M. D.**
Ultrasound Laboratory
Gentofte Hospital, University of Copenhagen
2820 Gentofte, Copenhagen
Denmark

**Tage Justesen, M. D.**
Associate Professor
Institute of Medical Microbiology
University of Copenhagen
Juliane Maries Vej 22
2100 Copenhagen
Denmark

**Per Ib Jørgensen, M. D., Ph. D.**
Chief Physician, Department of Gynecology
and Obstetrics
Herlev Hospital, University of Copenhagen
2730 Herlev, Copenhagen
Denmark

**Jørgen Kvist Kristensen, M. D., Ph. D.**
Chief Surgeon, Department of Surgery D
Section of Urology
Rigshospitalet, University of Copenhagen
Blegdamsvej 9, 2100 Copenhagen
Denmark

**Jørgen Falck Larsen, M. D., Ph. D.**
Professor, Department of Gynecology and
Obstetrics
Herlev Hospital, University of Copenhagen
2730 Herlev, Copenhagen
Denmark

**Svend Larsen, M. D.**
Department of Pathological Anatomy
Herlev Hospital, University of Copenhagen
2730 Herlev, Copenhagen
Denmark

**Hans van der Maase, M. D.**
Department of Onchology and Radiotherapy
Herlev Hospital, University of Copenhagen
2730 Herlev, Copenhagen
Denmark

**Hirochi Ohe, M. D.**
Department of Urology, Kyoto Prefectural
University of Medicine
Kawaramachi-Hirokoji, Kamigyo-Ku
Kyoto, Japan 602

**Jan Fog Pedersen, M. D.**
Director of Ultrasound Laboratory
Glostrup Hospital, University of Copenhagen
2600 Glostrup, Copenhagen
Denmark

**Poul Hjortkjær Pedersen, M. D.**
Chief Physician, Department of Gynecology
and Obstetrics
Herlev Hospital, University of Copenhagen
2730 Herlev, Copenhagen
Denmark

**John Philip, M. D., Ph. D.**
Professor, Department of Gynecology and
Obstetrics YA
Rigshospitalet, University of Copenhagen
Blegdamsvej 9, 2100 Copenhagen
Denmark

**Sten Nørby Rasmussen, M. D., Ph. D.**
Department of Medical Gastroenterology P
Rigshospitalet, University of Copenhagen
Blegdamsvej 9, 2100 Copenhagen
Denmark

**Masahito Saitoh, M. D.**
Department of Urology, Kyoto Prefectural
University of Medicine
Kawaramachi-Hirokoji, Kamigyo-Ku
Kyoto, Japan 602

**Edward H. Smith, M. D.**
Professor of Radiology
Peter Bent Brigham Hospital and
Sidney Farber Cancer Center
Harvard Medical School
44 Binney Street
Boston, Massachusetts 02115, USA

**Mogens Vilien, M. D.**
Department of Pathological Anatomy
Herlev Hospital, University of Copenhagen
2730 Herlev, Copenhagen
Denmark

**Hiroki Watanabe, M. D.**
Professor, Department of Urology
Kyoto Prefectural
University of Medicine
Kawaramachi-Hirokoji, Kamigyo-Ku
Kyoto, Japan 602

# Preface

When first adopted, the ultrasonically guided percutaneous puncture technique becomes quite indispensable in many clinical situations since it is virtually without risk and allows for easy and precise diagnostic or therapeutic contact with any ultrasonically visualized target.

It is the aim of this book to thoroughly describe the various ultrasonically guided puncture techniques, point out the many present applications, state results, discuss advantages and limitations including risks and also suggest possible future applications.

At the ultrasonic laboratory of Gentofte, now Herlev, Hospital, the first percutaneous puncture guided by ultrasonic scanning using a specifically designed transducer was performed in 1969. The idea was based on a puncture transducer described and used by Kratochwill for puncture under the guidance of the A-presentation technique.

In 1978 the Danish Society of Diagnostic Ultrasound sponsored the First International Conference on Ultrasonically Guided Puncture at Herlev Hospital. The great interest in the field demonstrated at this meeting and the ever-increasing use and spread of the method have suggested the need for a textbook on the subject. On this background, most of the speakers at the conference have agreed to record the knowledge and experience of their specific fields in individual chapters in this book.

We would like to acknowledge the excellent collaboration with all the contributors, which greatly facilitated the editing of the book.

Copenhagen, May 1980

H. H. Holm   J. Kvist Kristensen

# Contents

# CHAPTER I

# Abdominal ultrasound anatomy and pathology

Edward H. Smith

The utility of ultrasonically guided needle placement can be illustrated with the following case: A 54-year-old male saw his physician because of headache and fullness and swelling of the face. A chest x-ray revealed a right paratracheal mass adjacent to the right hilum. An ultrasound examination of the liver revealed a single lesion in the region of the caudate lobe of the liver (Figs. 1.1A and 1.1B). A clinical diagnosis of probable oat cell carcinoma of the lung with superior vena caval obstruction was considered likely but tissue diagnosis had to be obtained prior to institution of therapy. Instead of a thoracotomy or mediastinoscopy to obtain tissue from the mass itself, an ultrasonically guided fine needle aspiration of the liver lesion was carried out, revealing small cell carcinoma (Fig. 1.2) and therapy was promptly instituted.

Before focusing upon the applications of this technique, it is incumbent upon us to review the cross-sectional anatomy, first with cadaver sections and then correlating them with the normal abdominal structures. Some of the normal anatomic structures which may occasionally be confused with abdominal masses or other abdominal pathology will then be demonstrated. Finally, ultrasound appearance of representative masses which might be suitable for ultrasonically guided puncture will be reviewed.

A transverse section through the upper abdomen of a cadaver is illustrated in Fig. 1.3. The characteristic shape of the right lobe of the liver in cross-section is shown as well as that of the left kidney, spleen tip, and stomach in the left upper quadrant. The abdominal aorta just anterior to the vertebral body and the inferior vena cava are also characteristic landmarks. The portal venous branching is noted in the hilum of the liver. The section illustrated is taken cephalad to the level of the pancreas. The transverse section illustrated in Fig. 1.4 is taken several centimeters below Fig. 1.3 through the celiac axis, placing it at approximately the T12–L1 level. A transverse ultrasound section through approximately the same level from a normal person is paired with this cadaver section. In both the cadaver section and the comparable ultrasound section we see both the right and left lobes of the liver, the gall bladder, both kidneys on either side of the vertebral body, the abdominal aorta giving rise to the celiac axis, including the hepatic artery. The inferior vena cava is again

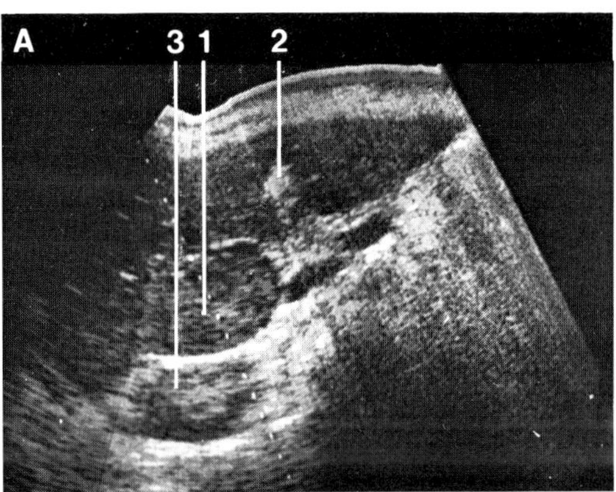

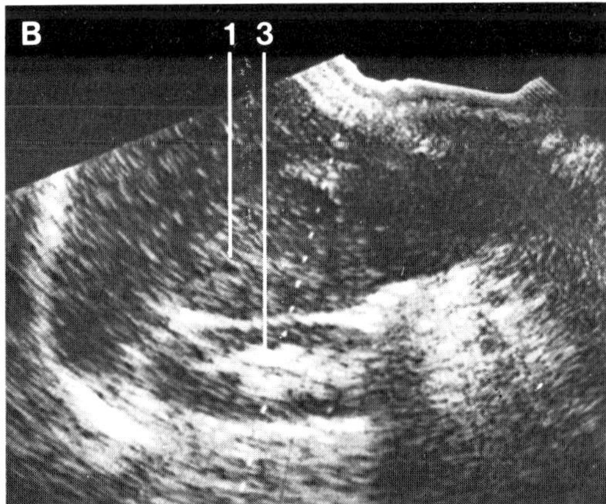

Fig. 1.1. *Liver metastasis*
A. Transverse scan through liver.
B. Longitudinal scan through liver.
1. Liver metastasis in caudate lobe. 2. Falciform ligament. 3. Right kidney. Dotted line is centimeter scale.

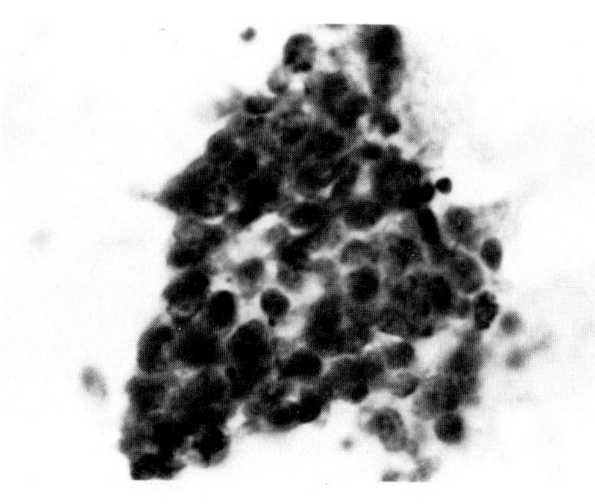

Fig. 1.2. *Cytologic aspirate*
Small cell carcinoma; aspirate from liver metastasis illustrated in Fig. 1.

seen. Anterior to the left kidney, best seen on the cadaver section, but also on the ultrasound section, is a portion of the tail of the pancreas. Just anterior to the pancreas is the stomach and colon. On the ultrasound section, these structures are filled with gas and thus obscure a portion of the pancreatic tail. In Fig. 1.5, the main portion of the pancreas is illustrated, both on cadaver section and on transverse ultrasound section. On both sections is a very useful landmark, the superior mesenteric artery, seen in cross-section as a small circular structure lying between the abdominal aorta and the body of the pancreas. The pancreas is seen to lie just below the left lobe of the liver. Somewhat further caudally in Fig. 1.6, a portion of body and head of the pancreas with the splenic vein lying between the body of the pancreas and the superior mesenteric artery is seen both on cadaver and ultrasound sections. Just to the right of the head of the pancreas is the duodenal loop on the cadaver section. On the ultrasound section, this landmark is seen as a rounded echo-poor structure with dense central echoes, the characteristic ultrasonic configuration of partially collapsed bowel. It is important not to confuse this structure with a mass or cyst when it is filled with fluid. In the slightly more cephalad ultrasound section (Fig. 1.6B), only a small portion of the splenic vein is seen along with the body and tail of the pancreas. A longitudinal section through the long axis of the inferior vena cava is illustrated in

Fig. 1.7. Hepatic veins emptying into the vena cava as well as the characteristic appearance of the portal vein in cross-section just anterior to the vena cava are well shown.

The normal ultrasonic architecture of the liver is shown in Fig. 1.8. The echo pattern is somewhat coarse with the typical appearance of normal hepatic venous branching. In contrast with the orderly echo pattern of the internal architecture of the liver, are the sharply defined echo-poor areas with centrally increased echoes seen in Fig. 1.9, representing liver metastases. Liver metastases may be either small or large, sharply defined or ill defined, echo-rich or echo-poor or any combination of these in any one patient. In general, however, most metastatic adenocarcinomas of the liver are echo-rich. Often it is difficult to distinguish among the various causes of echo-free focal liver lesions (Figs. 1.10, 1.11, and 1.12).

Cystic metastases may be from any primary malignancy, but most often are from sarcomas, frequently leiomyosarcoma. In the area of the liver in the region of the junction of the left and right lobes, a seemingly focal area of increased echogenicity is often visualized (Fig. 1.13). A computed tomographic scan of this area (in a different patient) reveals this to be the falciform ligament (Fig. 1.14). The ligament contains a variable amount of fat which is probably responsible for the ultrasonic appearance. It is important not to mistake this structure for a liver metastasis for obvious reasons.

As was stated earlier, the pancreas is a variably shaped structure, usually extending obliquely across the abdomen with the tail of the pancreas in the region of the hilum of the spleen and the head lying somewhat more caudally, bordered laterally by the descending duodenum. The pancreas lies beneath the left lobe of the liver and usually can be easily separated from it (Fig. 1.15). The splenic vein courses transversely along the posterior surface of the pancreas to join the superior mesenteric vein forming the portal vein. With acute pancreatitis the organ often becomes diffusely enlarged and somewhat more sonolucent due to edema (Fig. 1.16). Focal enlargement of the pancreas (Fig. 1.17) is more suspicious for a neoplasm. However, not every solid structure in the area is a malignancy of the pancreas. The caudate lobe of the liver often superficially has the appearance of a solid mass in the head of the pancreas

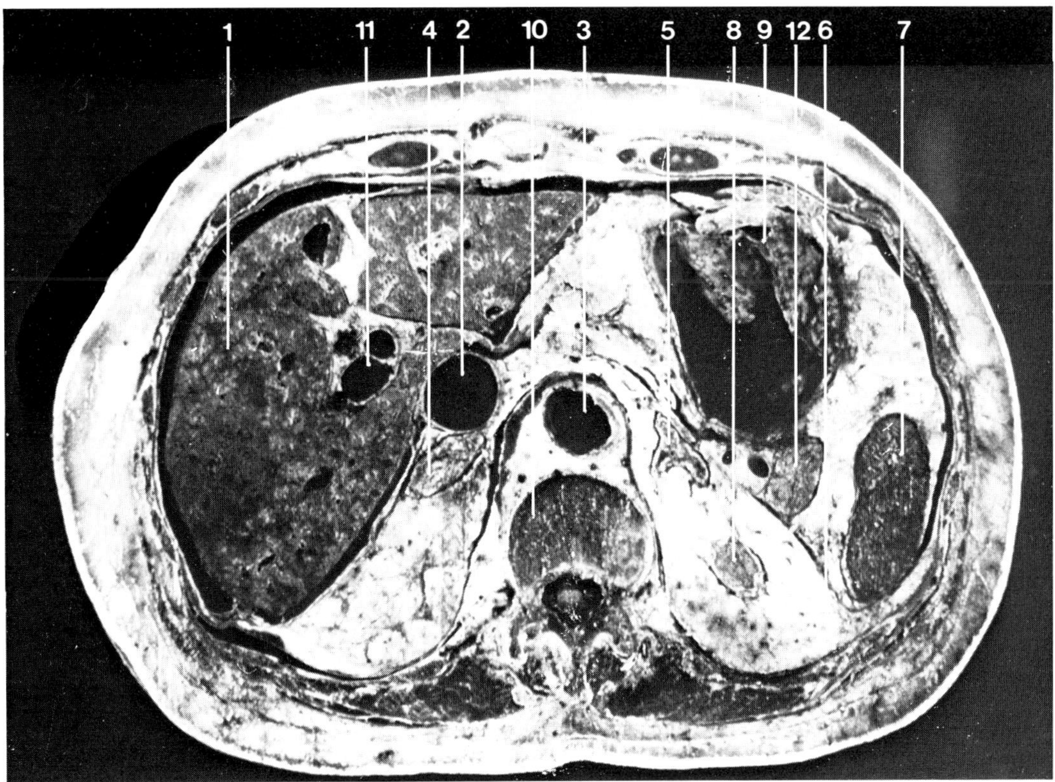

Fig. 1.3. *Cadaver section*
Transverse section through upper abdomen.
1. Liver. 2. Inferior vena cava. 3. Aorta. 4. Right adrenal. 5. Left adrenal. 6. Retroperitoneal fat. 7. Spleen tip. 8. Tip upper pole left kidney. 9. Stomach. 10. Vertebral body. 11. Portal vein bifurcation. 12. Pancreatic tail.

(Fig. 1.18), but careful scanning reveals the area to be contiguous with the liver and has the same ultrasonic architecture as normal liver. Stool in the splenic flexure may simulate a mass in the tail of the pancreas (Fig. 1.19). However, in this instance, repeat examination the same day after a bowel movement reveals the mass to have disappeared. A sharply defined cystic structure in the region of the pancreas in the proper clinical setting often leaves little doubt as to the presence of a pancreatic pseudocyst. If a fluid-debris level is seen, this is even further evidence in favor of the diagnosis (Fig. 1.20). However, one must be aware that a fluid-filled stomach may occasionally simulate a pseudocyst. The characteristic configuration of a fluid-filled stomach is shown in Fig. 1.21. If the patient is given a glass of fresh tap water, multiple small echoes can often be seen forming within the fluid due to the micro-bubbles in the water. This observation is facilitated by having access to a dynamic scanner.

Acute cholecystitis may be simulated clinically by an abscess in the vicinity of the gall bladder. An example of this is shown in Fig. 1.22, where an abscess is situated subcutaneously just superficial to the tip of the liver lying directly over the gall bladder. Ultrasound examination revealed the abscess and a normal gall bladder.

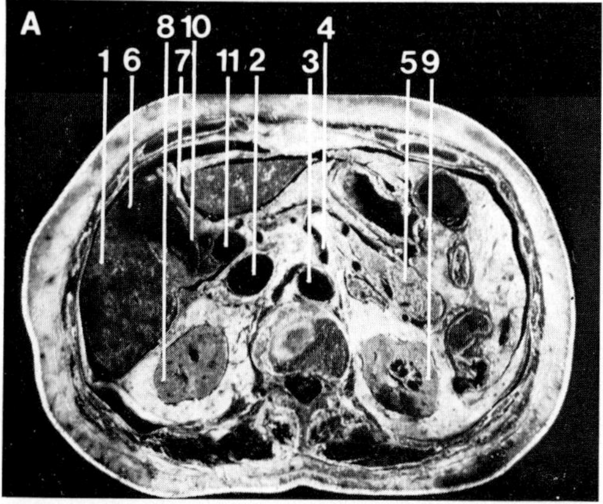

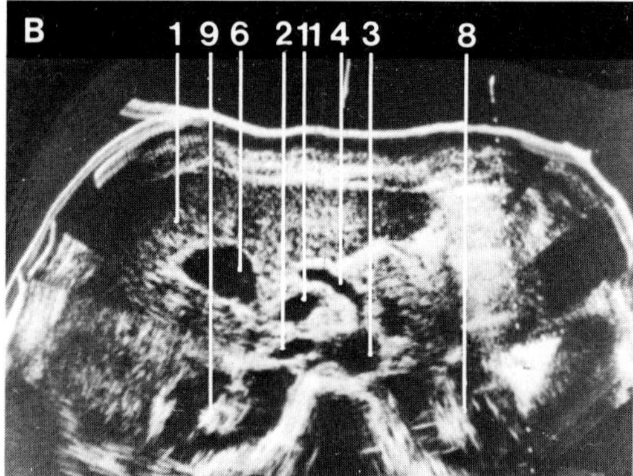

Fig. 1.4. *Cadaver and ultrasound section*
Transverse section slightly caudad to Fig. 3 through celiac axis.
A. Cadaver section.
B. Ultrasound section (living subject).
1. Liver. 2. Inferior vena cava. 3. Aorta. 4. Celiac axis. 5. Tail of pancreas. 6. Gallbladder. 7. Falciform ligament. 8. Left Kidney. 9. Right kidney. 10. Common bile duct. 11. Portal vein.

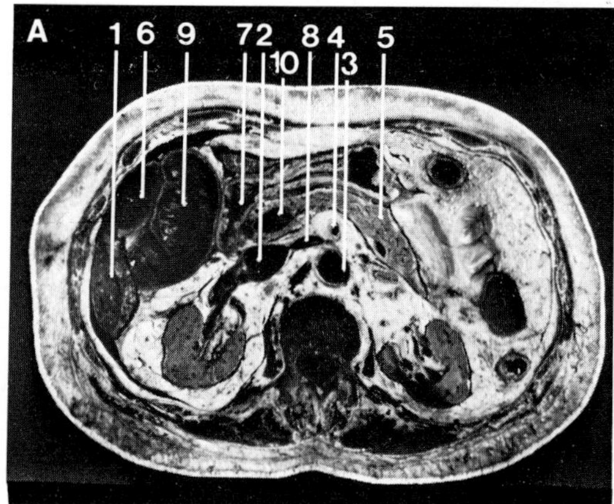

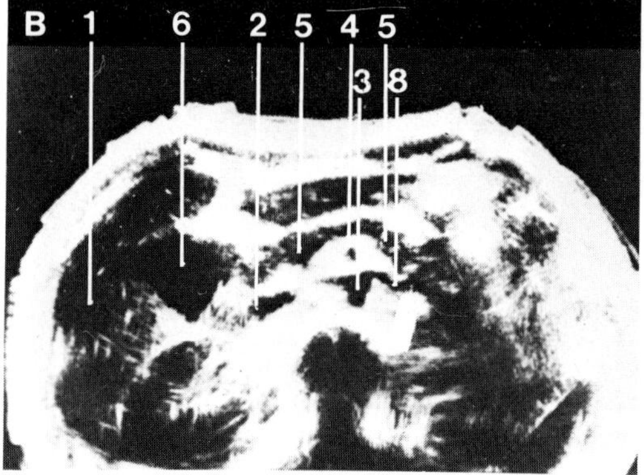

Fig. 1.5. *Cadaver and ultrasound section*
Transverse section caudad to Fig. 4 through body of pancreas.
A. Cadaver section.
B. Ultrasound section (living subject).
1. Liver tip. 2. Inferior vena cava. 3. Aorta. 4. Superior mesenteric artery. 5. Body and tail of pancreas. 6. Gallbladder. 7. Duodenum. 8. Left renal vein. 9. Hepatic flexure. 10. Superior mesenteric vein.

On longitudinal section, the normal common bile duct may be occasionally visualized ultrasonically. It courses anterior to the portal vein, seen on the cross section, to dip posteriorly through the pancreas toward its duodenal insertion (Fig. 1.23). Its final posterior course differentiates it from the hepatic artery, which turns to its origin in the celiac axis. A dilated duct usually does not present a diagnostic problem (Fig. 1.24).

The distinction between renal cyst and renal tumor usually offers no significant problem either. It is important in any work-up of a renal mass, however, that the search not be ended after a mass is discovered. Extent of the tumor must be carefully documented. In other words, the opposite kidney must be examined carefully for evidence of bilateral involvement. Retroperitoneal nodes must be excluded and the liver must be carefully



Anatomy and pathology

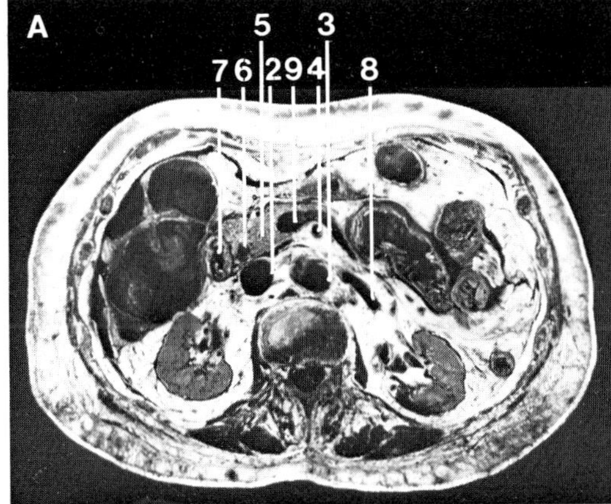
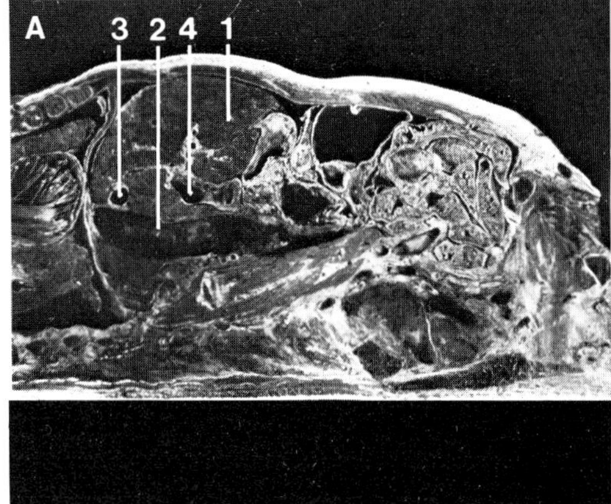
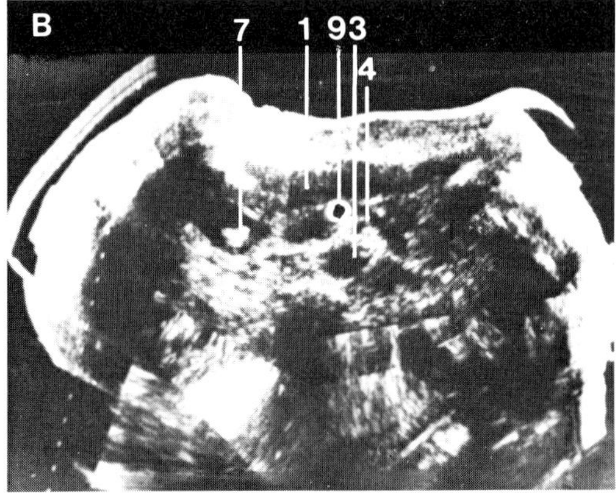
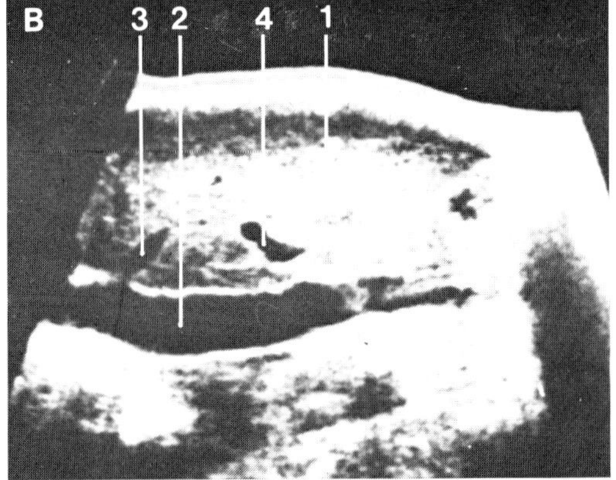

Fig. 1.6. *Cadaver and ultrasound section*
Transverse section caudad to Fig. 5 through head of pancreas.
A. Cadaver section.
B. Ultrasound section (living subject).
1. Left lobe of liver. 2. Inferior vena cava. 3. Aorta. 4. Superior mesenteric artery. 5. Head of pancreas. 6. Common bile duct. 7. Duodenum. 8. Left renal vein. 9. Splenic vein.

Fig. 1.7. *Cadaver and ultrasound section*
Longitudinal section through inferior vena cava.
A. Cadaver section.
B. Ultrasound section (living subject).
1. Liver. 2. Inferior vena cava. 3. Hepatic vein entering inferior vena cava. 4. Portal vein bifurcation in cross section.

examined for metastases (Fig. 1.25). In addition, the inferior vena cava must be carefully examined for evidence of tumor invasion (Fig. 1.26).

The term "suprarenal gland" really is a misnomer. especially when referring to the left adrenal gland. Tumors of the adrenal gland on the left usually lie central or anterior to the left kidney rather than above the left kidney (Fig. 1.27). In this patient with symptoms vaguely suggesting the possibility of a pheochromocytoma, excretory urography, nephrotomography and selective angiography all failed to reveal evidence of the tumor. Finally, because of the unequivocal ultrasonic findings, a repeat selective angiogram in the oblique position revealed the lesion. In the case of a suspected adrenal tumor it is important to attempt to delineate the border of the adjacent kidney in order to differentiate an adrenal tumor

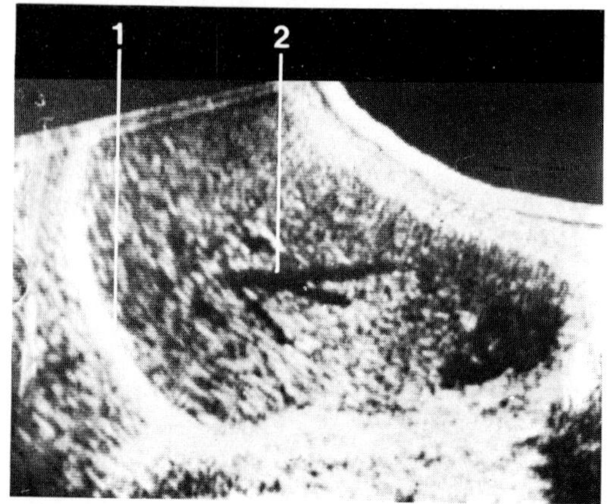

Fig. 1.8. *Normal liver*
Longitudinal section.
1. Diaphragm. 2. Hepatic venous branching.

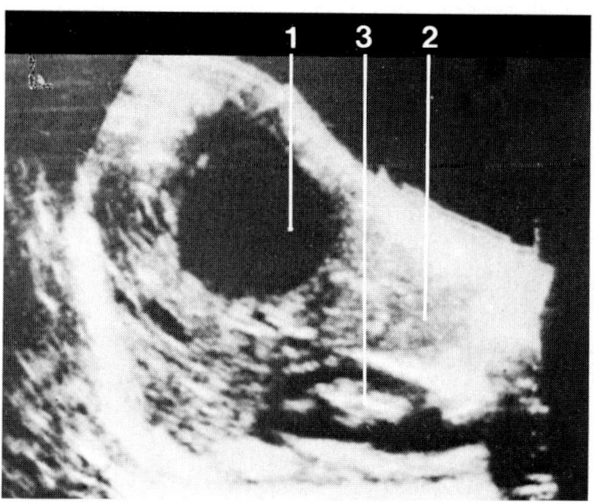

Fig. 1.10. *Liver abscess*
Longitudinal scan.
1. Echo-free abscess. 2. Normal liver. 3. Right kidney.

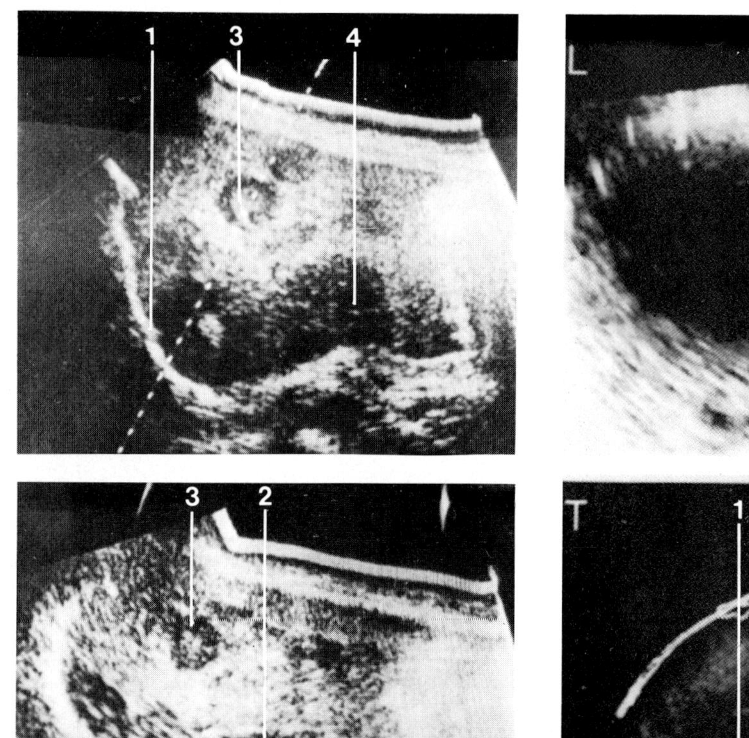

Fig. 1.9. *Liver metastases – "Target lesions"*
Two parallel longitudinal scans.
1. Diaphragm. 2. Right kidney. 3. "Target" metastases.
4. Confluent echo-poor metastases.

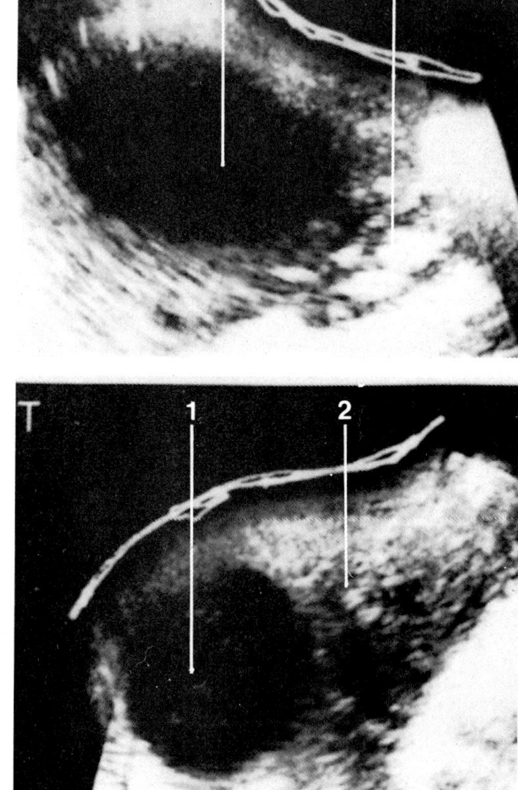

Fig. 1.11. *Liver hematoma*
Longitudinal (L) and transverse (T) scans.
1. Echo-poor hematoma. 2. Normal liver. 3. Right kidney.



Anatomy and pathology

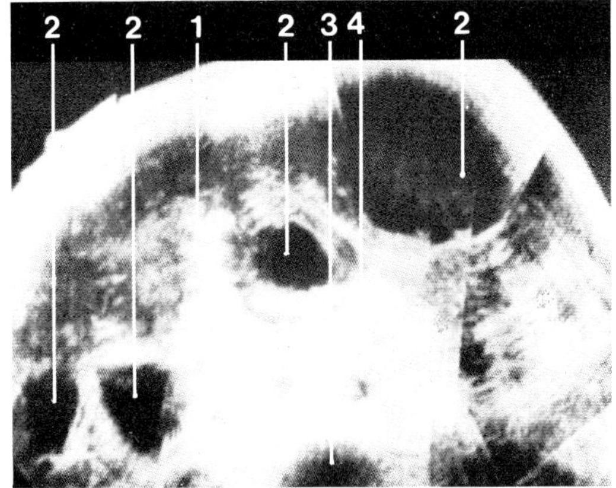

Fig. 1.12. *Liver metastases – Cystic*
Transverse scan.
1. Normal liver. 2. Echo-poor cystic metastases with thick rims. 3. Anterior tip of vertebral body. 4. Aorta. Primary lesion was leiomyosarcoma of the duodenum.

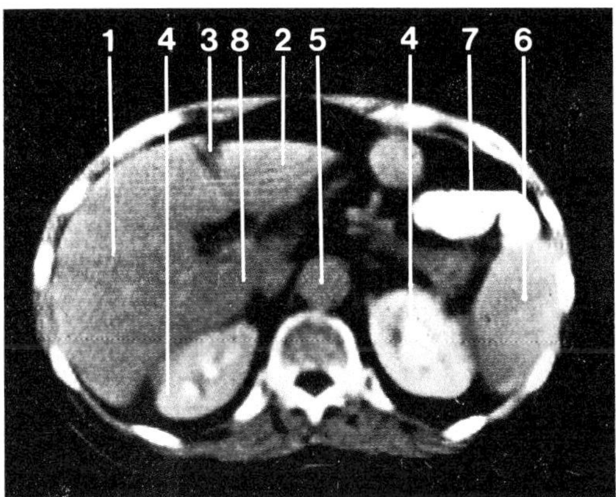

Fig. 1.14. *Falciform ligament*
Transverse computed tomogram.
1. Right lobe of liver. 2. Left lobe of liver. 3. Falciform ligament and surrounding fat. 4. Kidneys with contrast. 5. Aorta. 6. Spleen. 7. Contrast in GI tract. 8. Caudate lobe of liver.

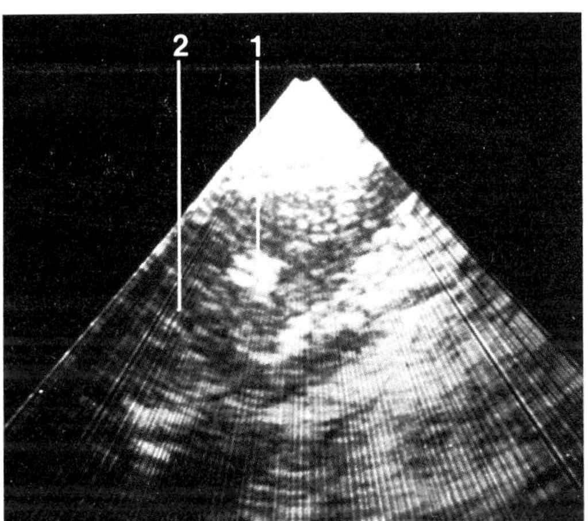

Fig. 1.13. *Falciform ligament*
Transverse dynamic sector scan.
1. Echo-rich "lesion" representing falciform ligament in cross-section mimicking a metastasis. 2. Normal liver.

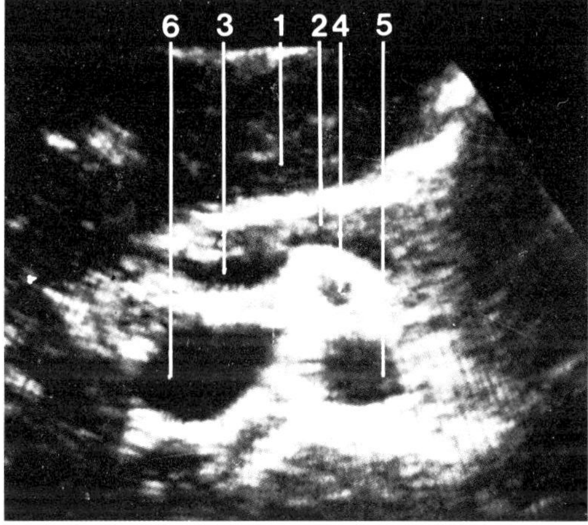

Fig. 1.15. *Normal pancreas*
Transverse scan – detailed view.
1. Left lobe of liver. 2. Body of pancreas. 3. Splenic vein. 4. Superior mesenteric artery. 5. Aorta. 6. Inferior vena cava. The normal pancreas is slightly more echogenic than the normal liver and contains coarser echoes.

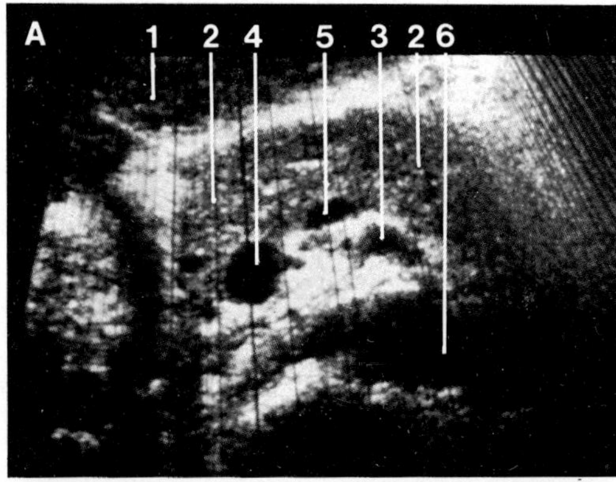

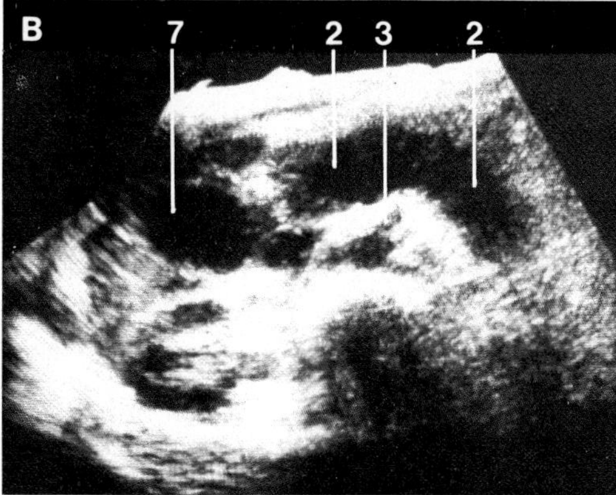

Fig. 1.16. *Acute pancreatitis*
A. Transverse scan – detailed view.
B. Transverse scan – second case.
1. Left lobe of liver. 2. Diffusely enlarged pancreas. 3. Superior mesenteric artery. 4. Superior mesenteric vein. 5. Portion of splenic vein. 6. Aorta. 7. Gallbladder.
Note that in "B" the pancreatic echoes are sparse and of low amplitude probably due to diffuse edema of the gland.

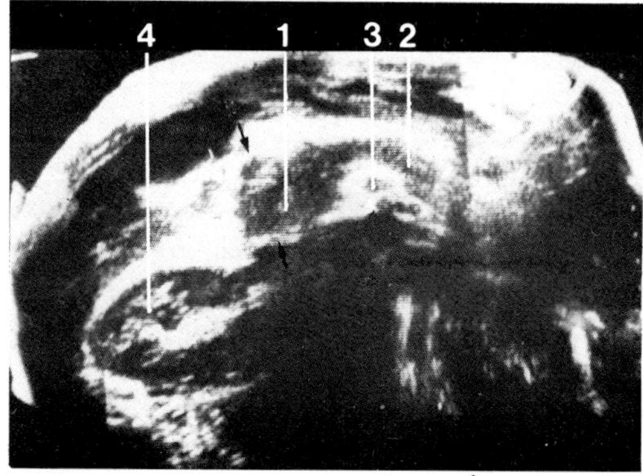

Fig. 1.17. *Carcinoma of the head of the pancreas*
Transverse scan.
1. Enlargement head of pancreas. 2. Normal body of pancreas. 3. Superior mesenteric artery. 4. Right kidney.

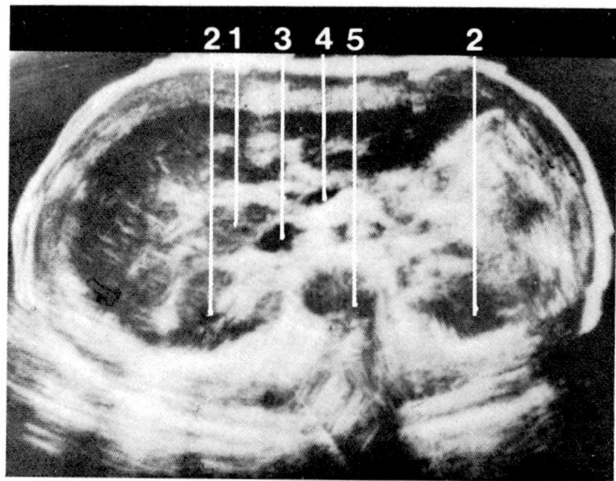

Fig. 1.18. *Caudate lobe of liver*
Transverse scan.
1. Caudate lobe of liver continuous with rest of liver. 2. Kidneys. 3. Inferior vena cava. 4. Splenic vein. 5. Vertebral body.

from a renal tumor (Fig. 1.28).

Ovarian cysts, when simple and unilocular, offer no diagnostic problem. However, when multilocular, it is almost impossible to be certain that a lesion is benign despite the presence of thin-walled septae. However, when the converse is the case, that is when the septae are irregularly thickened and nodular, then the lesion must be considered malignant until proven otherwise (Fig. 1.29).

Finally, to come full cycle, the utility of ultrasonic needle aspiration is illustrated with a brief case history. The patient in question had been operated on 4 weeks previously for carcinoma of the sigmoid colon. On routine physical examination, a moderate sized mass was palpable in the pelvis and the surgeon found it hard to believe that he had missed such a mass at surgery. He requested an ultrasonic examination which revealed an echo-poor but solid mass in the pelvis (Fig. 1.30). Again, because the surgeon could not believe that this mass represented a recurrence in so short a time period, percutaneous fine needle aspiration of the mass was carried out under ultrasound guidance. Microscopic examination under polarized light revealed starch crystals and the diagnosis of a starch granuloma was made and treated with steroids with rapid resolution, sparing both the patient and the surgeon a second operation (Fig. 1.31).



Anatomy and pathology

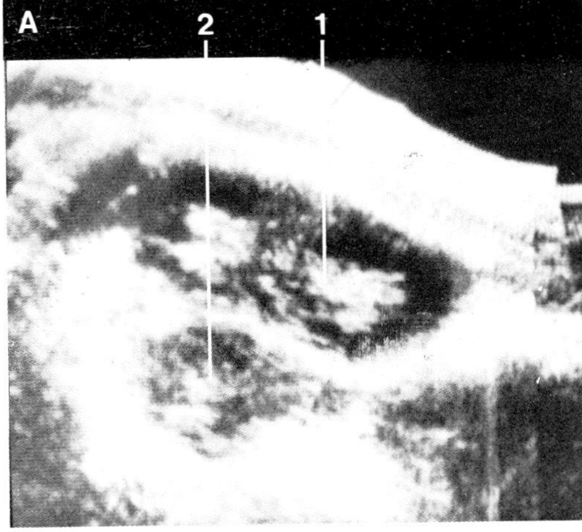

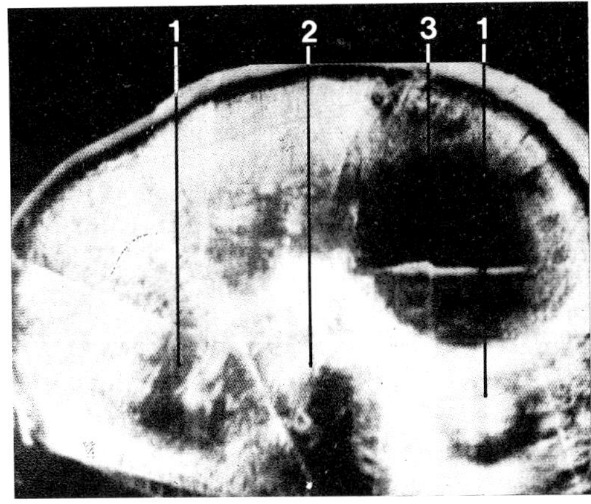

Fig. 1.20. *Pancreatic pseudocyst*
Transverse scan.
1. Kidneys. 2. Vertebral body. 3. Pancreatic pseudocyst with fluid-debris level.

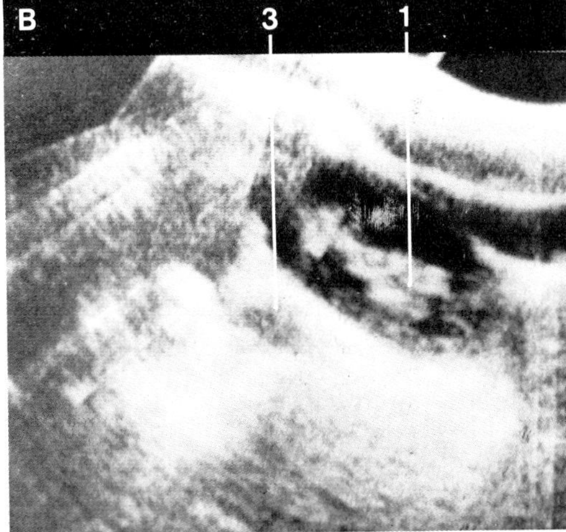

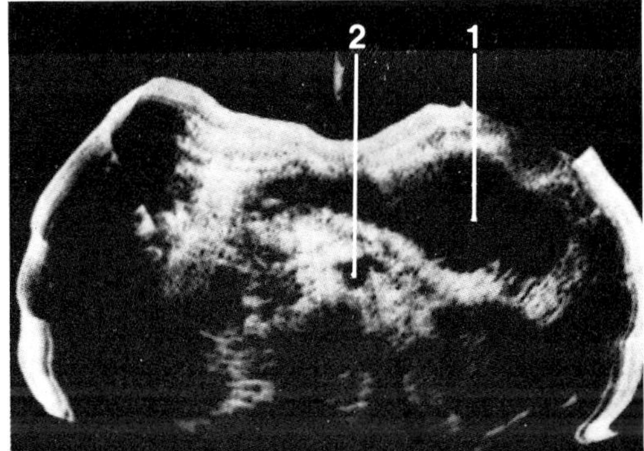

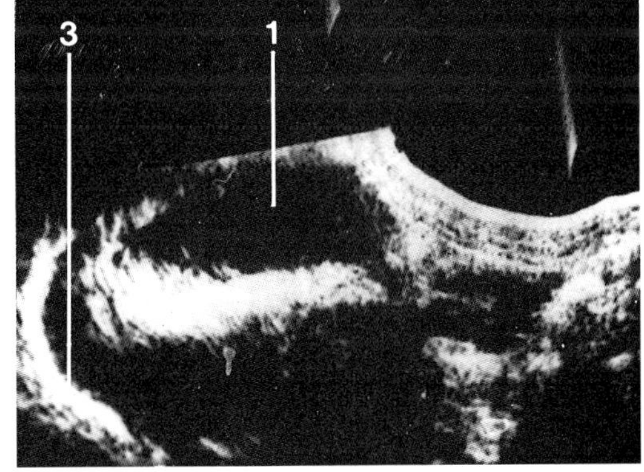

Fig. 1.19. *Stool in splenic flexure simulating carcinoma of tail of pancreas*
A. Longitudinal prone scan.
B. Longitudinal prone scan 3 hours later after colon evacuated
1. Left kidney. 2. ?mass in tail of pancreas. 3. Mass no longer present – normal colon.

Fig. 1.21. *Fluid-filled stomach*
Transverse (above) and longitudinal scans.
1. Fluid-filled stomach. 2. Aorta. 3. Diaphragm.
Note irregular strongly echogenic posterior wall on longitudinal scan, characteristic of stomach contents which is in contrast to sharp interface of the pancreatic pseudocyst in fig. 1.20.

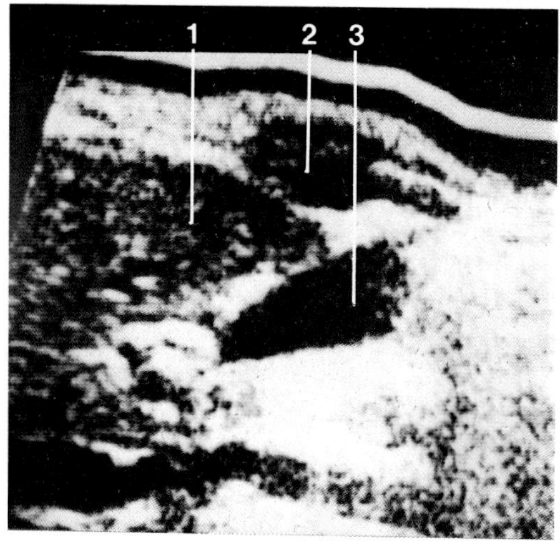

Fig. 1.22. *Abdominal wall abscess simulating acute cholecystitis*
Longitudinal Scan.
1. Inferior edge right lobe of liver. 2. Abdominal wall abscess. 3. Normal gallbladder.

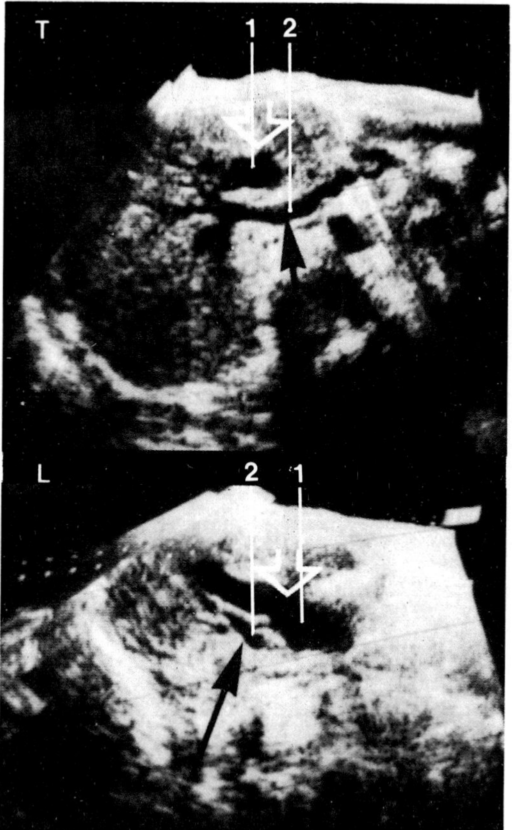

Fig. 1.24. *Dilated common bile duct*
Transverse (T) and Longitudinal (L) scans.
1. Markedly dilated common (hepatic) bile duct. 2. Portal vein. The bile ducts run anterior to the portal vein.

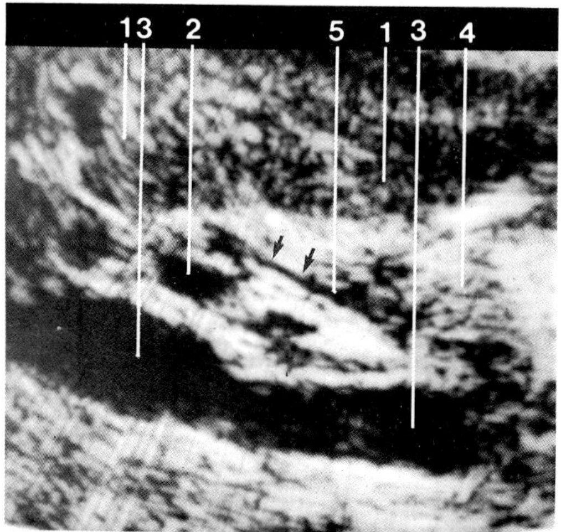

Fig. 1.23. *Normal common bile duct*
Longitudinal scan – detailed view.
1. Liver. 2. Portal vein. 3. Inferior vena cava. 4. Pancreas. 5. Common bile duct.



Anatomy and pathology

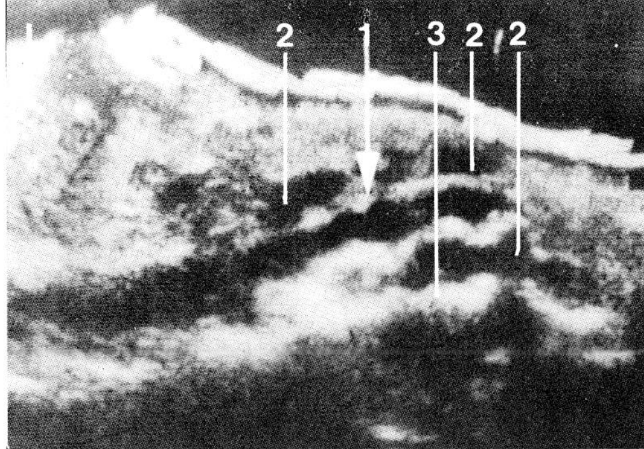

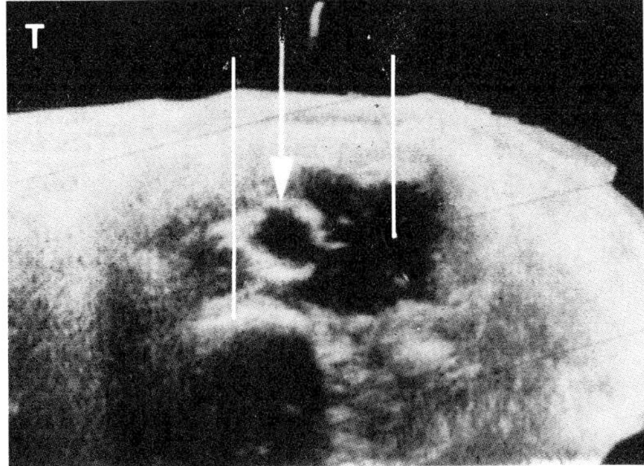

Fig. 1.25. *Retroperitoneal adenopathy*
Longitudinal (L) and Transverse (T) scans.
1. Aorta. 2. Metastatic paraaortic lymphadenopathy. 3.
Anterior vertebral body.
Adenopathy surrounds aorta and lifts it off the vertebral
body. In this particular example, the primary lesion is in
the prostate, rather than the kidney.

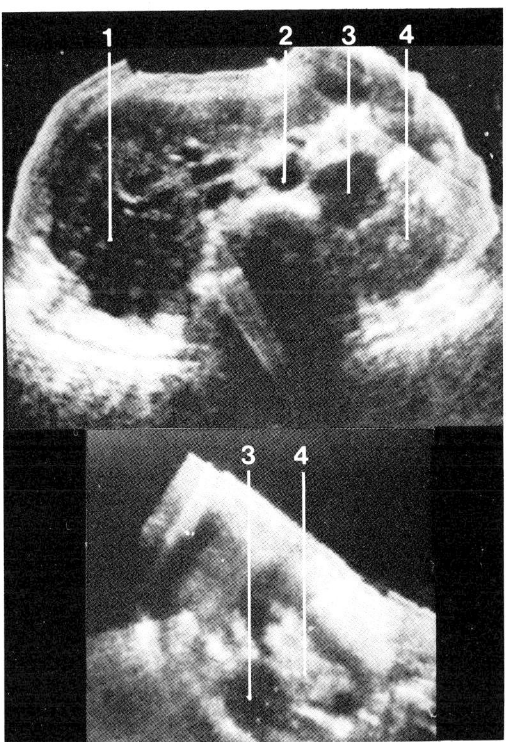

Fig. 1.27. *Pheochromocytoma*
Transverse supine (top) and longitudinal prone scans.
1. Liver. 2. Aorta. 3. Mass in left adrenal gland. 4. Left
kidney.

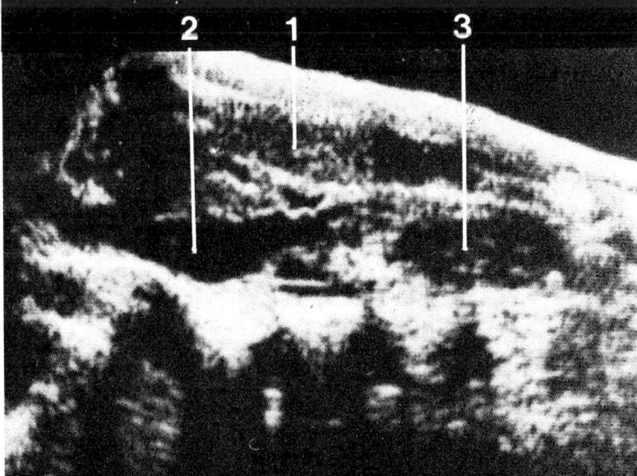

Fig. 1.26. *Renal carcinoma invading inferior vena cava*
Longitudinal scan.
1. Lever. 2. Inferior vena cava. 3. Tumor thrombus within
inferior vena cava.

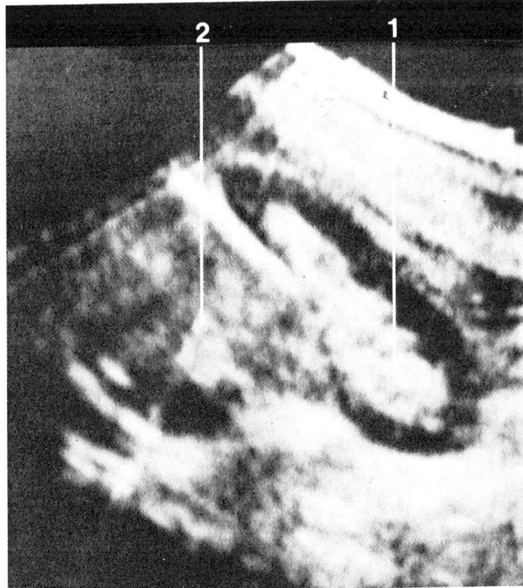

Fig. 1.28. *Adrenal tumor*
Longitudinal prone scan.
1. Left kidney. 2. Adrenal mass deforming left kidney.

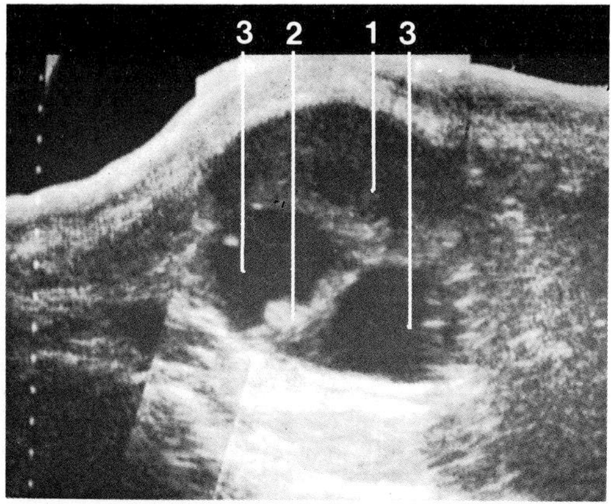

Fig. 1.29. *Ovarian cystadenocarcinoma*
Longitudinal scan – detailed view.
1. Complex ovarian mass. 2. Nodular, irregularly thickened septum. 3. Cystic component.

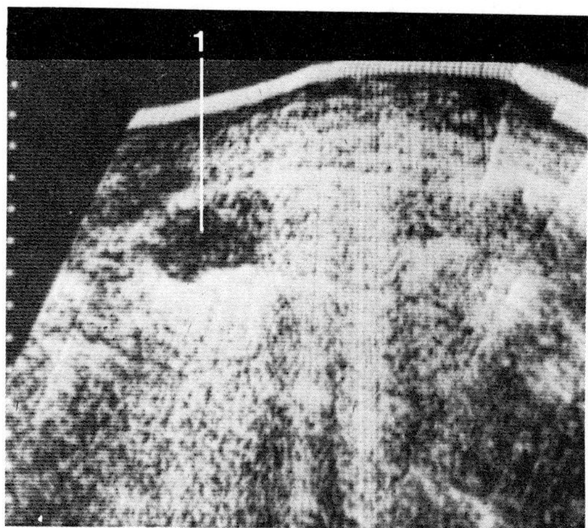

Fig. 1.31. *Starch granuloma after steroid therapy*
1. Echo-poor solid mass – marked reduction in size after two weeks of steroid therapy.

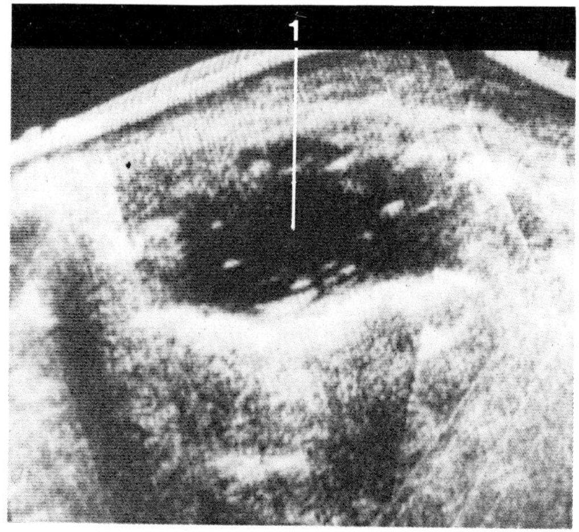

Fig. 1.30. *Starch granuloma*
Transverse scan through pelvis.
1. Echo-poor solid mass containing sparse, coarse echoes.

# References


Holm, H. H., Kristensen, J. K., Rasmussen, S. N., Pedersen, J. F., Hancke, S., Jensen, F., Gammelgaard, J. and Smith, E. H.: Abdominal Ultrasound, 2. edition. *Munksgaard*, Copenhagen, 1980.

# CHAPTER II

# Physical principles for ultrasonically guided puncture

Flemming Jensen

When a reliable diagnosis is to be made on the basis of a percutaneous biopsy, it is important that the sample is obtained precisely from the center or edges of the lesion as intented. This requires a method of meaningful visualization, so that the position, extent and possible nature of the lesion can be determined prior to the puncture. Ultrasonic scanning offers such possibilities.

Palpatory guidance of the sampling needle may be of value when puncturing superficial masses but has no place in the puncture of deeply situated masses.

Ultrasonic scanning is well suited for imaging of palpable as well as non-palpable masses, provided they are not completely obscured by air or bone, and it offers precise guidance of a needle to any visualized point of interest.

The basic principle of ultrasonically guided puncture is that with the use of a transducer with a central canal, a needle introduced through this canal will follow the direction of the sound beam which is visualized on the TV-monitor image (Fig. 2.1.). The beam is aimed at the target and the needle can be inserted to the correct depth.

Provided the tip is in an echo-free or echo-poor mass, an echo of medium amplitude is seen on the A-scope, corresponding to the depth of the tip (Fig. 2.2). This echo amplitude is a complex function of the diameter of the needle (see Chapter III).

It is not obvious why the needle tip is visualized on the A-scope. The needle tip does *not* represent an ordinary reflector more or less perpendicular to the sound beam. Goldberg and Ziskin have given the explanation that the echo production is due to reconstitution of the beam, after it has been disrupted by the length of the needle in the beam axis. The echo amplitude is in the order of magnitude of

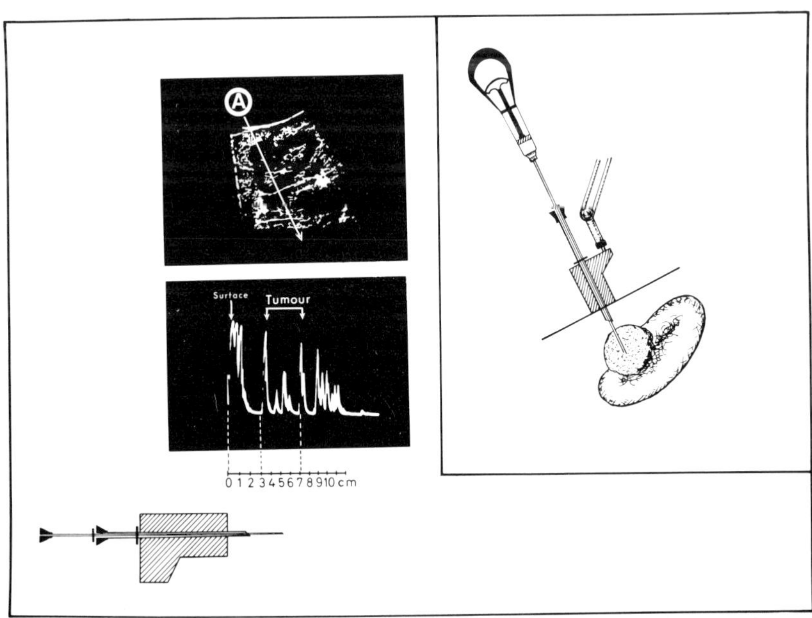


Fig. 2.1 *Ultrasonically guided puncture principle*
For explanation see text.

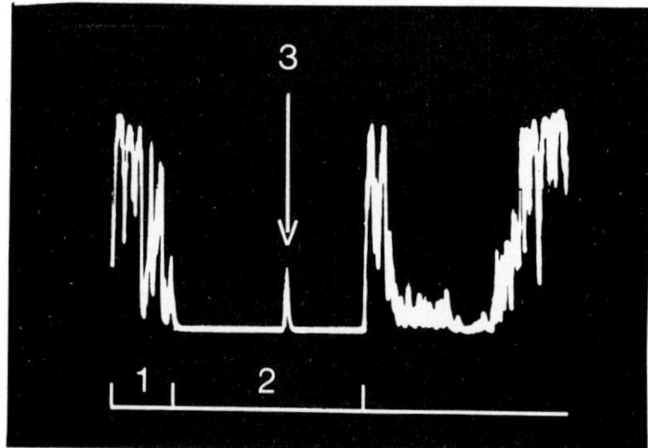

Fig. 2.2 *Needle tip echo*
A-mode presentation of the echo spike corresponding to the position of the needle tip (3) inside a cystic lesion (2). 1 indicates solid tissue.

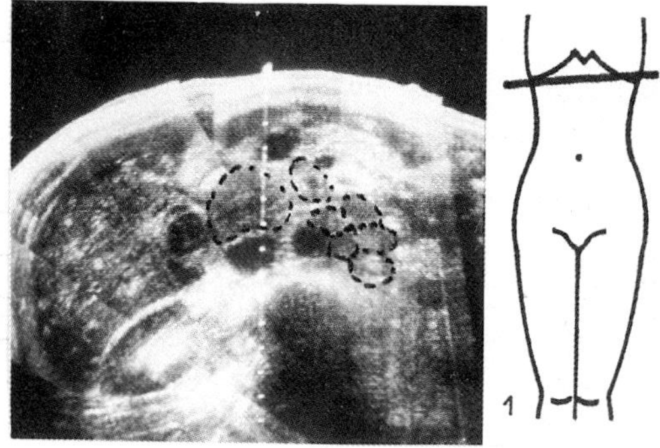

Fig. 2.3 *Electronic marker*
The dotted line superimposed on the B-mode image (i.e. an electronically generated centimeter-marker line) pointing towards the mass lesion to be punctured, in this case lymphomas in the upper retroperitoneal region.

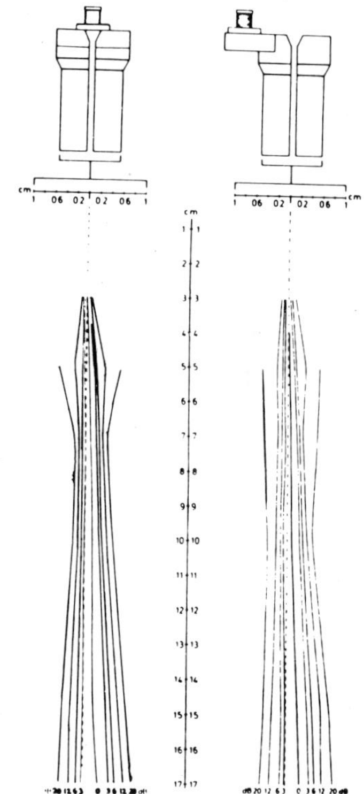

Fig. 2.4 *Ultrasonic beam pattern*
An isointensity plot of a puncture transducer. The beam profile is plotted in two perpendicular planes in the direction of the beam. Ideally the extension of the central canal in the transducer should be situated exactly in the beam axis.

echoes within many solid structures. Therefore the needle tip echo will be lost in the image of a solid tumor, while it will be clearly demonstrated in a cyst.

If the equipment is adjusted to an average sound velocity, f.ex. 1540 m per sec, which corresponds to the sound velocity in most tissues, then the exact depth of the needle tip is registered, enabling precise placement deep under the surface. Regarding non-cystic lesions to be punctured, one has to rely on the dotted electronic line which can be superimposed on a static B-mode image (Fig. 2.3). Aided by this marker-line, the proper depth can be measured and the *axial* accuracy of the puncture is secured.

The *lateral* accuracy in aiming with the electronic marker line depends on a number of factors:
1) that the transducer housing has an axis coinciding with the axis of the sound beam
2) that the scanner arm geometry (i.e. the rod system with angle sensors) is correctly adjusted in the image plane
3) that the "play" or flexibility of the arm perpendicular to the scanning plane is minimal.

To ensure that the introduced needle will travel along the dotted line on the image screen, which represents the intended needle path, a number of other requirements must be fulfilled:
1) The central canal in the puncture transducer shall have an axis common with the axis of the sound beam.
   On a commercially available transducer it has been shown that the deviation of these two



Physical principles

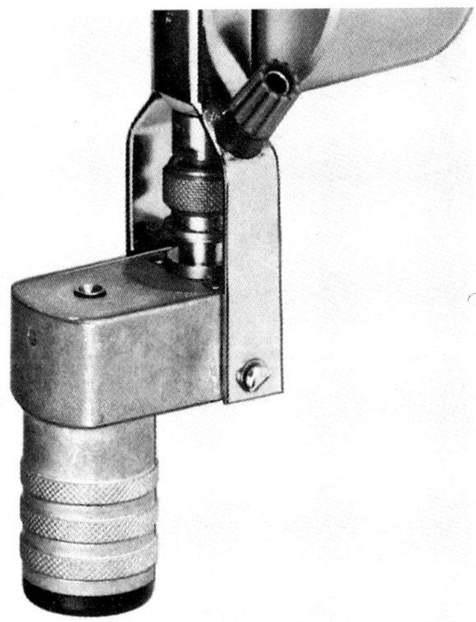

Fig. 2.5 *Adapter tube*
Adapter tube intended to steer the needle precisely in the axis of the canal in the puncture transducer.

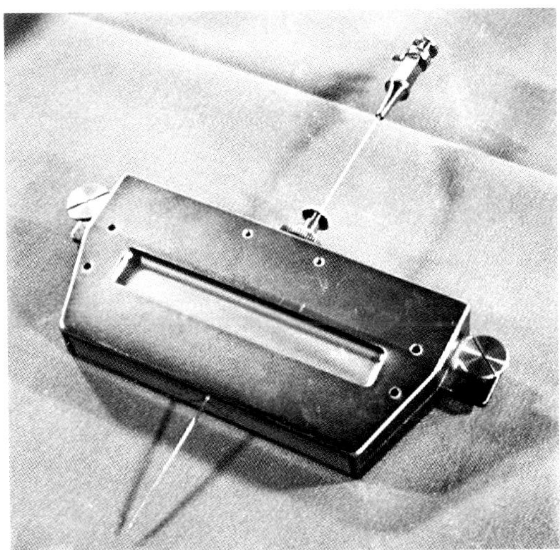

Fig. 2.7 *Dynamic scanning with direct needle introduction*
This multielement transducer has a central canal to steer the puncture needle parallel to the sound beams.

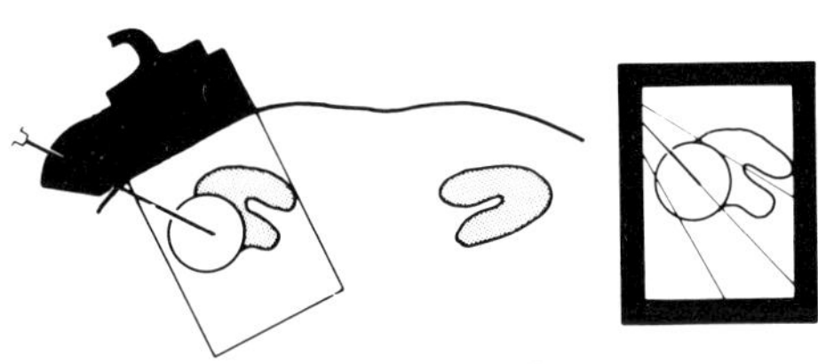

Fig. 2.6 *Dynamic scanning with oblique needle introduction*
The needle steering device on this prototype linear array scanner will secure introduction of the needle into the sound field in a predetermined angle with respect to the transducer face.

axes at a depth of 10 cm is approximately ± 2 mm (Fig. 2.4).

2) To steer the needle properly, the canal in the transducer must have a certain length, usually 4 to 6 cm (Fig. 2.5). With the use of thin needles, adapter tubes should be inserted to give the canal a diameter less than half a millimeter larger than the needle diameter. Thus the "play" of the needle will be acceptable.

The "play" has been shown to be approximately ± 5 mm at a depth of 10 cm with a commercially available transducer having a height of 6 cm.

3) Bending of the needle in the tissues may occur with standard fine needles having a diameter of 0.6 mm. Experiments on cadavers have shown that the orientation of the obliquely sharpened needle tip is without significance in this respect. Introduced into a depth of 8 cm in the flank of cadavers, X-ray control revealed bending of the fine needle to a maximum of 5 mm.

The above-mentioned factors, which in combination tend to diminish the accuracy in ultrasonic puncture, all have a physical or technological background.

Major factors may be organ movements in the patient and improper needle introduction by a less experienced examiner. Also sound beam refraction will theoretically be of some significance even in soft tissues. This is the only problem which in practice is beyond any control, as it is uninfluenced by examiner experience and equipment quality.

In some situations puncture monitored by a dynamic scanner can be advantageous, but it is ideal in cases with small constantly moving targets. Until now mainly electronic linear array transducers with some sort of needle steering device have been available:

1) The needle may be introduced obliquely into the sound field (Fig. 2.6).

2) The needle may follow a canal centrally in the array of transducer elements (Fig. 2.7). In this case one transducer element in the array is replaced by the canal, but nevertheless in cysts the needle tip is seen in the image lines of the neighboring elements. This may be due to some beam broadening from the small single elements, to the limited electrical insulation between the elements or the multiplexed activation of the elements, or a combination of these factors.

Whatever the explanation, experience has shown that such a transducer is most useful, especially in amniocentesis.

## References

Goldberg, B. B. and Ziskin, M. C.: Echo patterns with an aspiration ultrasonic transducer. *Invest. Radiol.* 8:78, 1973.

Holm, H. H., Kristensen, J. K., Rasmussen, S. N., Northeved, A. and Barlebo, H.: Ultrasound as a guide in percutaneous puncture technique. *Ultrasonics* 10:83, 1972.

Pedersen, J. F.: Percutaneous puncture guided by ultrasonic multitransducer scanning. *J. Clin. Ultrasound* 5:175, 1977.

# CHAPTER III

# Puncture needles and ultrasonic wave propagation in ultrasonically guided puncture

Hans-Erik Hjelmroth

Two main physical problems are involved in ultrasonically guided puncture: 1) the determination of the exact position of the puncture target, and 2) the determination of the position of the needle tip.

The solution of these problems is rather difficult since it is not easy to established well-defined experimental conditions which relate resonably well to the clinical situation.

## INFLUENCE OF TISSUES ON ULTRASONIC IMAGING

When a sound beam traverses the abdomen, it will pass numerous interfaces between tissues with different sound velocities. Thus human tissues may form various types of "refracting elements", which can be divided into two principally different types, the planar and the wedge shaped (Fig. 3.1).

In some cases also lense-shaped refracting elements may occur. Such refracting elements give rise to transverse as well as longitudinal distortions of the ultrasonic beam.

## Experimental investigations

The ultrasonic field of a centro symmetric ultrasonic puncture transducer was recorded in a water tank with 0.9% saline by measuring the reflections from a mechanically scanned 3-mm steel ball placed at various distances from the transducer and at various distances from the central axis of the transducer. The signal was displayed on spark-sensitive paper quantitated in three levels of intensity. Pieces of pig's belly flesh were then placed in front of the transducer with new recording of the ultrasonic field. As illustrated in Fig. 3.2, diffraction and focusing of the

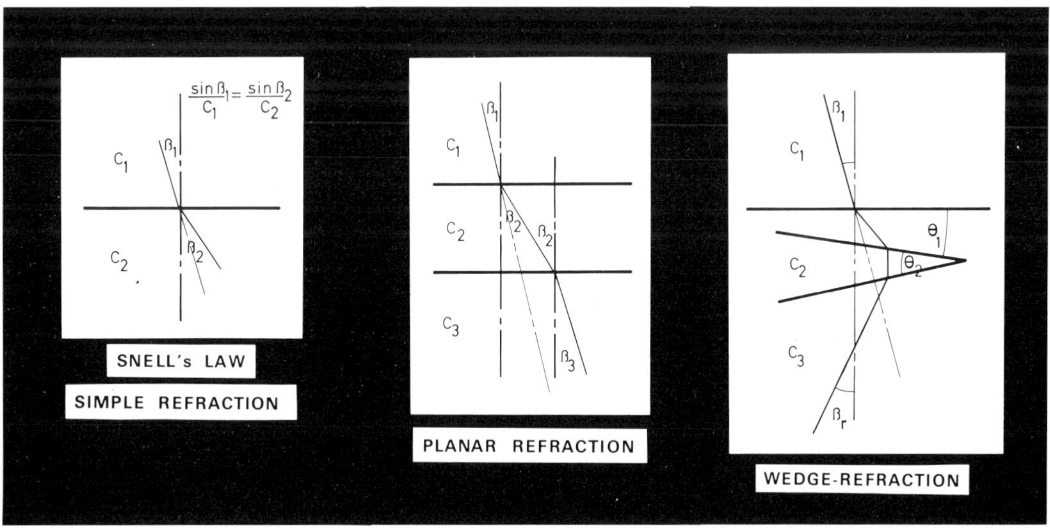


Fig. 3.1. *Refraction elements*
Refracting elements, schematically illustrated in this figure, cause displacement of the ultrasonic beam everywhere in the human body.

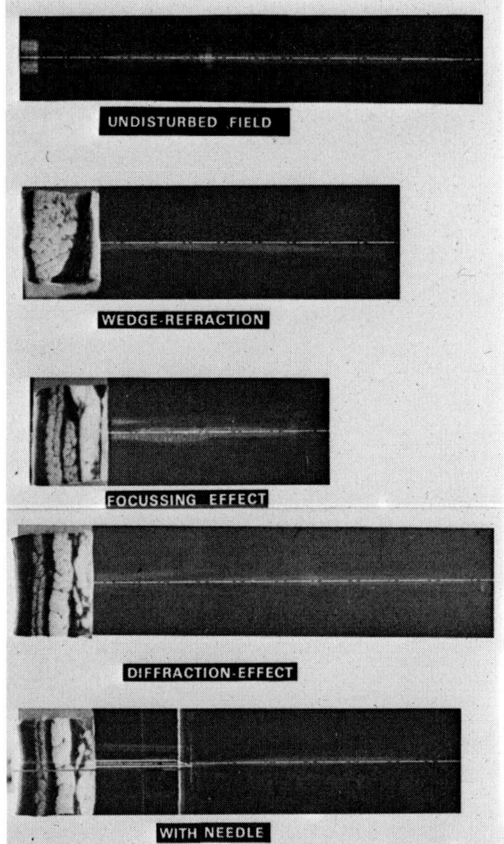


Fig. 3.2. *Distortion of the sound field during simulated abdominal scanning*
The sound field from a puncture transducer was experimentally measured. At top, the undisturbed field followed by various types of refraction and diffraction caused by pieces of pig's belly flesh. At bottom, the influence of an inserted needle is registered.

ultrasonic beam may be produced. The possible influence of a needle in the diffracted ultrasonic field was in an order of magnitude not recordable in the experimental set-up.

## Clinical implications

As the amount of various tissue types and their shape vary individually it is not at present possible to perform a correction for the distortion of the ultrasonic field in a clinical situation.

The transverse distortion, for example, may be of some relevance when a kidney is scanned in a linear fashion and this is schematically shown in Fig. 3.3. It appears that when the sound beam hits the oblique muscle-fat interface posterior to the

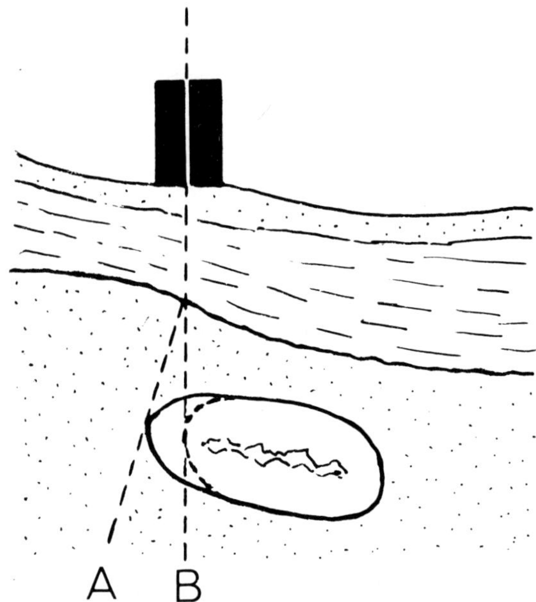


Fig. 3.3. *Result of ultrasonic field distortion*
In this schematic example, diffraction of the beam occurs when it hits the oblique muscle-fat interface posterior to the kidney. This results in a decrease of the length of the kidney on the image. A, real projection, B, ultrasonic projection.

upper renal pole, a diffraction occurs which tends to decrease the length of the kidney on the image. An estimate of the degree of distortion can be obtained by compairing a linear and a compound scan of the same area.

## CHANGES OF THE ULTRASONIC FIELD CAUSED BY THE PUNCTURE NEEDLE

Usually the longitudinal position (the depth) of the tip of the needle is easily determined in fluid-filled cavities.

In solid structures, however, the needle tip signal has the tendency to drown in the signals, diffracted and reflected from the surrounding structures.

In this case an improvement of the signal-to-noise ratio is needed especially for the needles with a diameter less than a wave length of the applied ultrasound. In practice this means needles with diameters less than 0.6 mm.

Goldberg & Ziskin (1973) found an overall increase of the intensity of the reflected/diffracted



Ultrasonic wave propagation

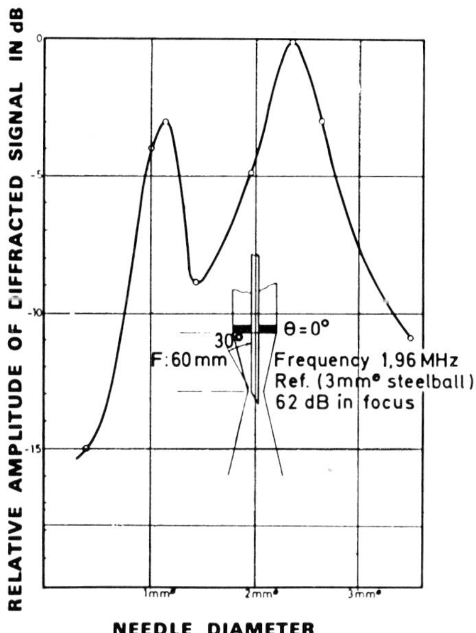



Fig. 3.4. *Needle tip signal as a function of needle diameter*

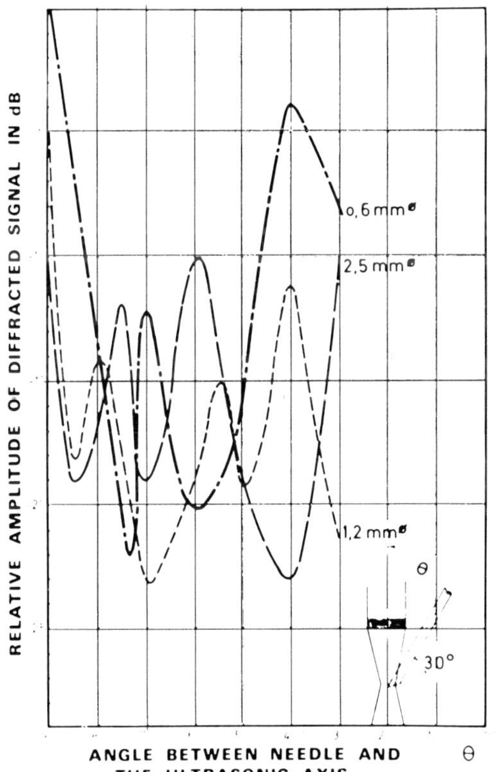



Fig. 3.5. *Needle tip signal as a function of the angle between the ultrasonic field axis and the axis of the needles for different diameters of needles*

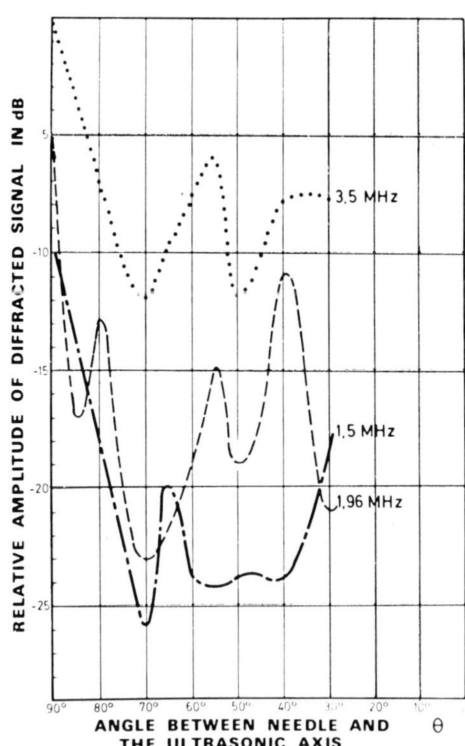



Fig. 3.6. *Needle tip signal as a function of the angle between the ultrasonic field axis and the axis of the needles for different frequencies*

ultrasonic signal from the needle tip with an increase in needle diameter.

## Experimental investigations

The interaction between ultrasonic fields of different frequencies and needles of different diameters and sharpness, as well as the influence of the angle between the ultrasonic field and the needle axis, have been investigated.

When various sized needles were introduced into the focal point through a 1.96 MHz puncture transducer, the needle tip signal as a function of the needle diameter was obtained. It is demonstrated that the response of the ultrasonic field to the presence of the needle tip is of the diffraction type rather than being due to pure reflection. This is clearly demonstrated in Fig. 3.4 in which the two resonances at 1.2 and 2.4 mm in needle diameter for 1.96 MHz indicate that the needle tip is resonantly diffracting the ultrasonic field.

Figs 3.5 and 3.6 show the needle tip signal as a

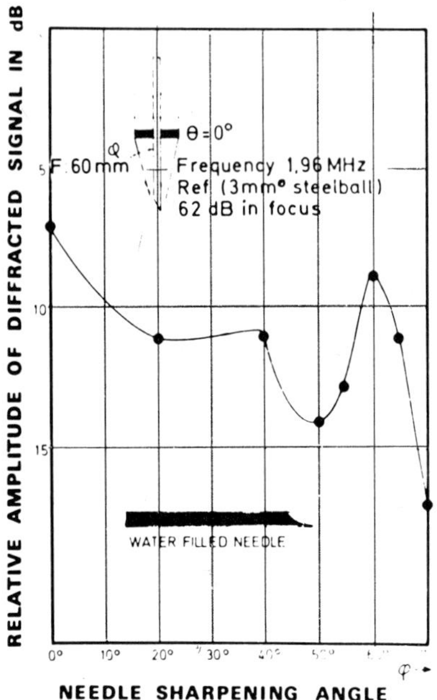


Fig. 3.7. *Needle tip signal as a function of the sharpening angle of the needle tip*

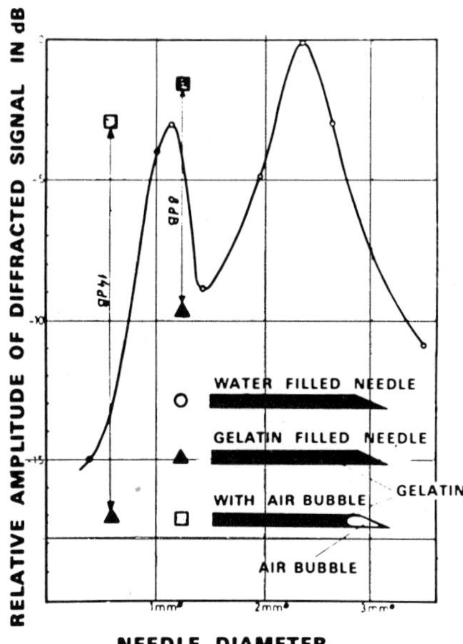


Fig. 3.8. *Needle tip signal from needle containing small air bubble compaired to signals from needles filled with water and gelatine, respectively*

function of the angle between the ultrasonic field and the needle axis for different diameters of the needles and different transducer frequencies, respectively. Characteristic intensity peaks of the resonantly diffracting target are apparent.

The needle tip signal is relatively independent of the sharpening angle of the needle except in the zero and high (70°) degree regions, where the signal is relatively strong and weak, respectively (Fig. 3.7). Both are of rather limited interest from a practical point of view.

In an effort to increase the needle tip signal, various procedures have been attempted.

The presence of acoustically low impedance materials in the needle point, as for example in the form of an air bubble, was attempted in a 1.2 and a 0.6 mm needle and gave rise to a considerable increase in the needle tip response (Fig. 3.8).

A more practical method would be to use needles which are macro-etched in the needle tip region (Fig. 3.9). Preliminary results suggest that an increase of about 15 dB in the needle tip signal can be obtained.

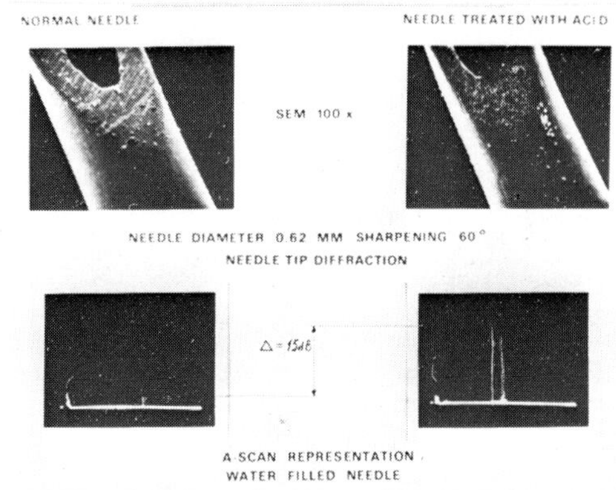


Fig. 3.9. *Macro-etching of needle tip and result on needle tip signal*
Scanning electron microscopy shows the significant change of the surface from smooth with small cracks from the drawing to a longitudinal row structure.

# References


Goldberg, B. B. & Ziskin, M. C.: Echo patterns with an aspiration ultrasonic transducer. *Invest. Radiol.* 8:78, 1973.

# CHAPTER IV

# Procedure of ultrasonically guided puncture

Hans Henrik Holm

Ultrasound can in many cases disclose an abdominal abnormality but frequently not provide information about the exact nature of the lesion.

Currently much research is carried out in the field of "tissue characterization" by means of ultrasound. Such characterization which may be based on frequency analysis of the returned echoes or on damping or velocity measurements is fascinating and will probably prove most valuable, e.g. in the diagnosis of diffuse liver disease or in the evaluation of the content of a fluid-filled process.

However, it is not likely that such methods or CT-scanning will be able to differentiate between benign and malignant lesions, to demonstrate the presence of bacteria, chromosome abnormalities, etc.

Therefore, also in the future there will in a great number of cases be a need for a more direct diagnostic approach in combination with abdominal ultrasound.

Furthermore, there will in many cases be a need for some kind of therapeutic procedure related to or directed against the ultrasonically demonstrated pathology.

Direct diagnostic or therapeutic contact with the structures visualized ultrasonically can easily, precisely and virtually without risk in most cases be obtained by means of an ultrasonically guided puncture.

In its simplest form, such a puncture is performed only on the basis of the ultrasonic scanning picture. From the scans the optimum site, direction and depth of the puncture are estimated. In most cases, however, it is advantageous to carry out the puncture while actually visualizing the target in question. Special equipment is required for this purpose.

## EQUIPMENT AND PROCEDURE

### Puncture guided by static scanning

The puncture is performed using a special puncture transducer, which is the same as an ordinary transducer except for a central canal through which a needle may be introduced (Fig. 4.1). The needle follows the direction of the sound beam and consequently can be guided into the target on the basis of the image and the sound direction indicator on the monitor (Fig. 4.2).

To allow room for needle manipulation, the connector of the transducer is displaced off-axis by means of a short horizontal bar. Adapters for the central canal are available, allowing the use of various sized needles.

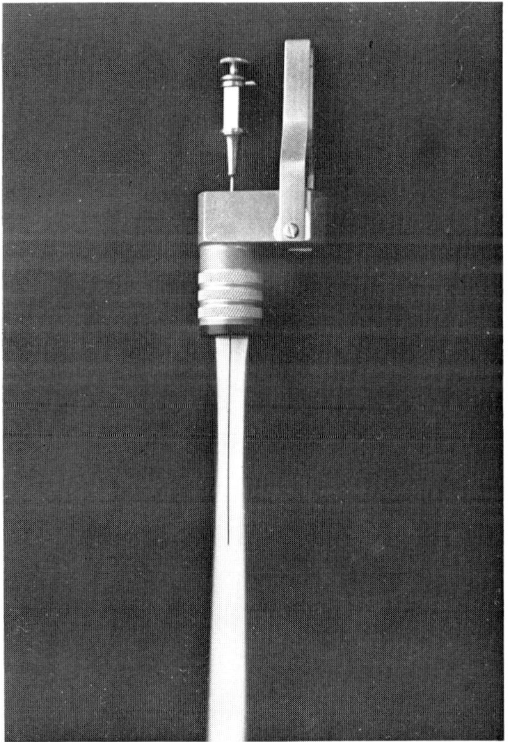

Fig. 4.1. *Puncture transducer*
The transducer is displaced off axis and has a central canal through which needles may be inserted. The needle will follow the sound beam emitted from the transducer.

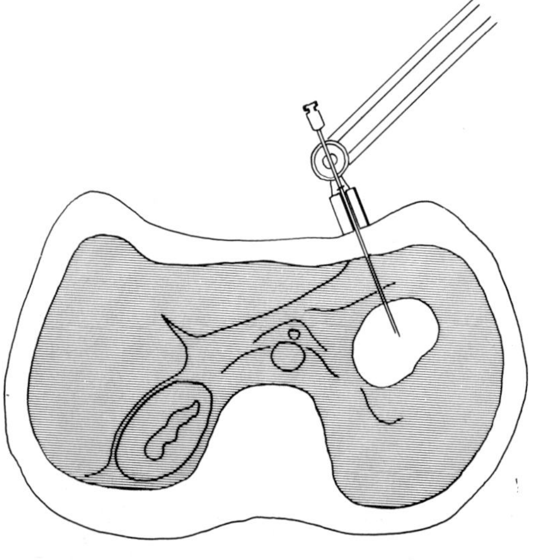

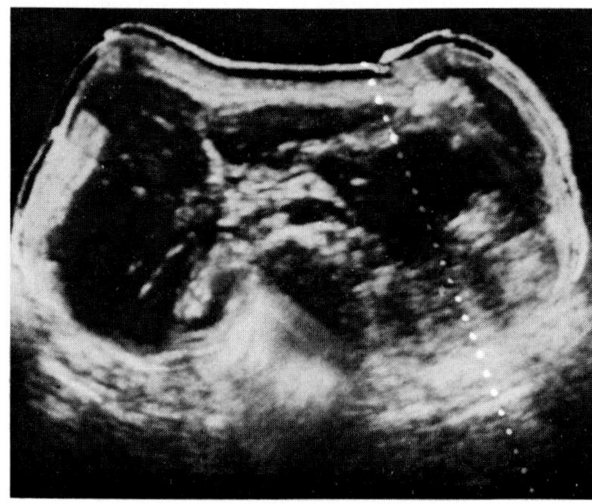

Fig. 4.2. *Principle of ultrasonically guided puncture*
The puncture target is visualized on a scan. On the basis of the scan and the sound direction indicator the optimum puncture site and direction are determined. The distance from the skin to the center of the target plus the length of the transducer are marked on the needle which is then inserted.

When routine examination has disclosed a puncture target, the puncture is suggested to the referring clinician and in case of liver and pancreatic punctures, bleeding time and coagulation time are required. Large needle liver and kidney biopsies require 500 cc of blood in the bank. In all other cases no preparations are taken except informing the patient.

When the puncture has been decided, the optimum plane and direction of puncture are selected. The shortest puncture distance is nor-

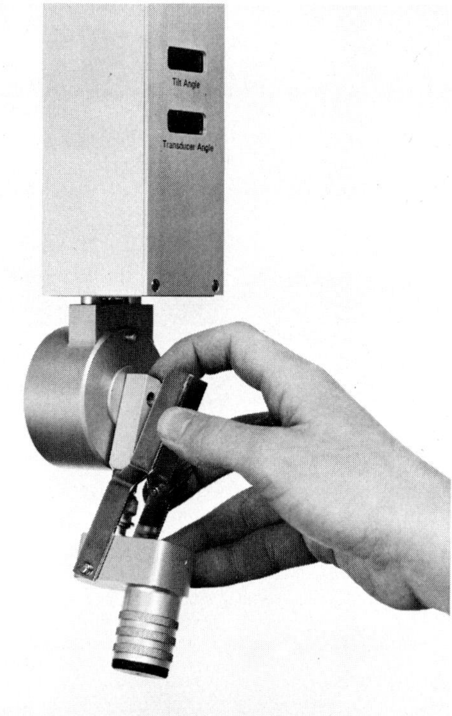

Fig. 4.3. *The puncture transducer is mounted on the scanning arm*

mally chosen not least because precision is thereby increased. This means, for instance, that kidneys are always punctured from the back.

Hundreds of punctures performed through the gastrointestinal tract and many through the urinary bladder have in our laboratory proved to be safe.

Because of the slight risk of minor liver lacerations with subsequent bleeding following transhepatic puncture, this route is omitted if possible.

However, if for instance a pancreas is not accessible without transhepatic puncture, such puncture is performed without hesitation.

Obviously, puncture through the pleura should be avoided. It means for instance that upper pole renal lesions should be punctured in a cephalad direction.

The patient should be asked to avoid extensive respiratory movements during the puncture and in some instances, e.g. when the puncture target is very small, it is an advantage to suspend respiration during the puncture.

Finally it is probably not wise to puncture le-



Puncture procedure

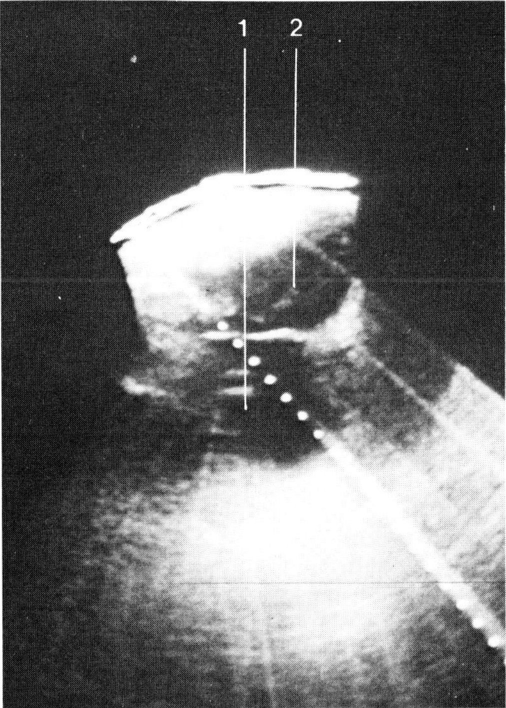

Fig. 4.4. *Fluid collection below lower pole of renal graft*
Transverse scan through right iliac fossa, supine position. 1. Fluid collection, 2. Lower pole of renal transplant. The marker indicates the optimal puncture route, avoiding puncture of the graft.

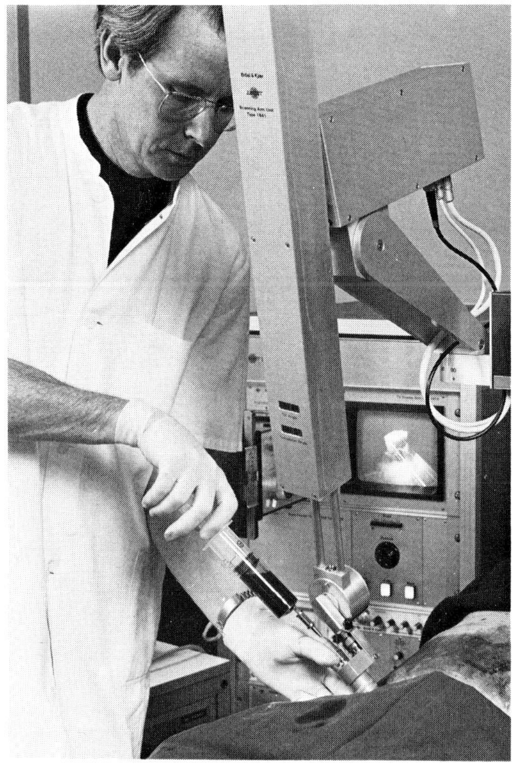

Fig. 4.5. *The aspiration is performed*
Using local anesthetic the puncture has been carried out through the puncture transducer guided by the image seen on the monitor in the background. A hematoma is aspirated.

sions suspected to be pheochromocytomas, ecchinococcus cysts or aneurysms.

If a fluid-filled target is suspected, the following technique is used: The site for the puncture is marked on the skin, which is then prepared and draped as for any sterile procedure. A local anesthetic is administered and sterile oil is applied to the skin.

The puncture transducer has been sterilized in chlorhexidine 0.5% in alcohol for 10 minutes or Korsolin[R] 3% in water for 30 minutes, the latter being effective against a broad spectrum of bacteria and virus including hepatitis. This can also be achieved by the use of glutaraldehyde 2% for 3 hours.

The puncture transducer is mounted on the scanning arm and the area of interest is rescanned using sterile oil (Fig. 4.3).

At the site previously marked, the puncture transducer is placed on the skin and angulated until the beam, visualized by the depth marker on the TV-monitor, coincides with the desired needle pathway (Fig. 4.4). The distance from the skin to the target is then measured on the scan. This distance plus the length of the puncture transducer are marked off on the needle. The needle is then introduced through the puncture transducer to the appropriate depth and the material aspirated – or the drugs injected (Fig. 4.5). If the lesion is echo-poor or echo-free, the tip of the needle can be seen on A-mode as a single strong echo which moves with the needle.

When a scanconverter is used, the echo from the needle does not appear on the "frozen" image and the tip of a fine needle is not registered at all.

This problem can be solved indirectly: On top of

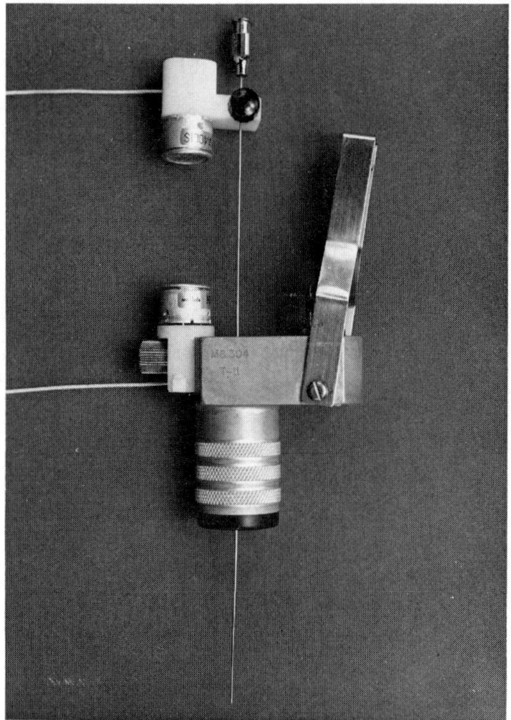

Fig. 4.6. *Needle tip indicator*
On top of the puncture transducer a small 40 KHz pulsating ultrasound transmitter is mounted. A corresponding receiver is fixed on the selected needle. A registration of the distance between these two points is thereby possible. A constant indication on the scan of the needle tip is thereby possible (see text).

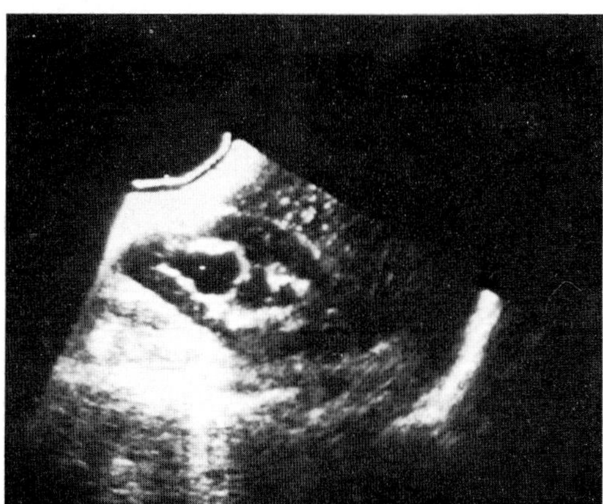

Fig. 4.7. *Needle tip indicated*

the ordinary puncture transducer a small 40 KHz pulsing ultrasound transmitter is placed and a corresponding receiver is fixed at the upper end of the needle in use (Fig. 4.6). Thereby precise distance measurements between these two points are

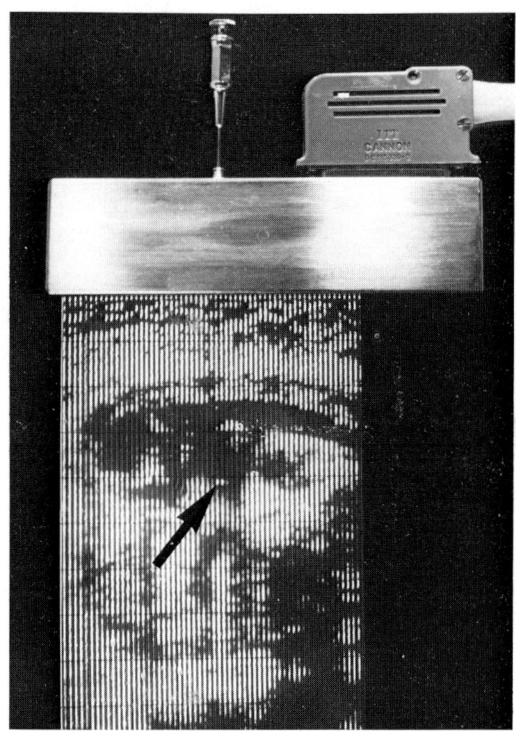

Fig. 4.8. *Puncture using dynamic scanning*
Composition showing multielement transducer equipped with puncture canal through which a needle is inserted into an amniotic cavity (early amniocentesis). The needle tip (arrow-marked) is visible.

possible. Prior to the puncture the needle is inserted in the puncture transducer with its tip at the level of the transducer front and the distance indicator is set at zero position by pressing a button. A flashing light dot on the scanconverter image indicates continuously the position of the tip when the needle is introduced (Fig. 4.7). The indicator is correct under the presumption that the needle docs not bend.

## Puncture guided by dynamic scanning

Puncture guidance by means of dynamic scanning has some obvious advantages. A moving target is visualized while the puncture is actually being performed. This may be valuable in amniocentesis when the fetus may move and also in renal biopsies (Fig. 4.8). Furthermore the whole needle or the needle tip may be visualized during the insertion. While dynamic scanners of the *electronic* type may

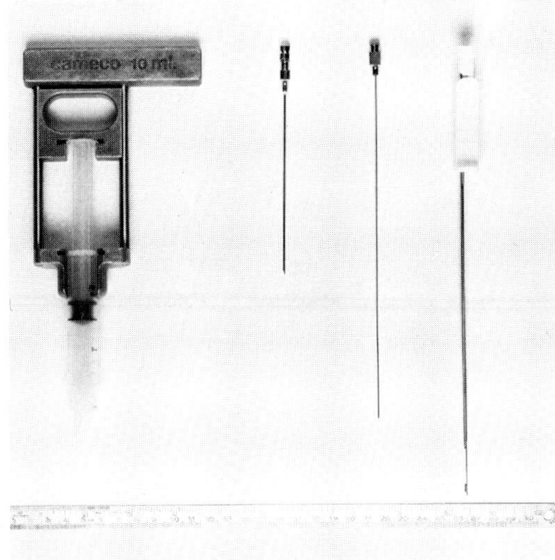

Fig. 4.9. *Puncture equipment*
A, Aspiration handle mounted with a 10cc syringe, B, 1.2 mm (18 gauge, lumbar) needle, C, 0.6 mm fine needle (23 gauge), D, coarse needle (Tru-cut®-type).

be equipped with a central puncture canal without problems, this can not for obvious reasons be done with a *mechanical* type such as a rotating transducer scanner. In these cases the puncture has to be performed obliquely into the sound field.

## Puncture needles

When the puncture target is supposed to contain fluid such as pus, blood, urine, etc., a 1.2-mm outer diameter so-called lumbar needle (18 gauge) is routinely used (Fig. 4.9). When a solid mass is suspected, a 0.6-mm (23 gauge) needle is used – as described in chapter V. A large bore cutting needle may be of the Tru-cut – or the Menghini type, for example.

## HAZARDS

Ultrasonically guided puncture has been carried out at the ultrasound laboratory at the Gentofte (now Herlev) Hospital since 1969. More than 2500 ultrasonically guided punctures of abdominal lesions have been performed. Clinically significant complications have been almost nonexistent. One patient after renal cyst puncture required a 1000-ml blood transfusion after a fall in hematocrit. In another patient with obstructive jaundice, puncture of a dilated gall bladder with subsequent injection of contrast (revealing obstructing common duct calculi) caused a 500-ml bile leak requiring immediate surgery.

There have been no instances of infection or fistula formation.

Of all cases undergoing ultrasonically guided needle aspiration subsequently operated upon, three hematomas at the needle sites were incidentally noted. The three cases were all different – a pancreatic pseudocyst, an adrenal adenoma and a renal mass. It is of course not unusual to find punctate hemorrhage at the puncture site at surgery, but on the other hand the biopsy site is often not visible.

The possible risk of spreading tumor cells is of major importance when a biopsy of a suspected malignant lesion is performed. This theoretical risk will be discussed in chapter XXI.

Obviously the degree of discomfort in conjunction with the puncture varies very much from patient to patient and from one puncture type to another, and it is quite impossible to give any objective measure of the amount of discomfort. However, it is striking that most punctures carry little or no discomfort.

## References

Holm, H. H., Kristensen, J. K., Rasmussen, S. N., Northeved, A. and Barlebo, H.: Ultrasound as a guide in percutaneous puncture technique. *Ultrasonics* 10:83, 1972.

Holm, H. H., Pedersen, J. F., Kristensen, J. K., Rasmussen, S. N., Hancke, S. and Jensen, F.: Ultrasonically guided percutaneous puncture. *Radiol. Clin. North Am.* 13:493, 1975.

# CHAPTER V

# Procedure of ultrasonically guided fine needle aspiration biopsy

Jens Gammelgaard

In the evaluation of solid masses or questionable lesions, the fine needle aspiration biopsy technique using a 23-gauge needle (outer diameter 0.6 mm) is preferable. Percutaneous fine needle aspiration biopsy under ultrasonic guidance can be applied to any organ or mass lesion which can be identified on the ultrasound scan.

The procedure is simple to perform, expeditious, requires few preparations and precautions, and is associated with little discomfort to the patient.

## EQUIPMENT

For most purposes a manual compound B-scanner is advantageous since the transducer is kept in a constant plane by the scanning arm. This allows for repeated biopsies. Guidance by dynamic scanning may be advantageous in some cases. The biopsy target may be so big and easily palpable through the abdominal wall that the use of a biopsy transducer is superfluous.

Apart from a thin 23-gauge needle (outer

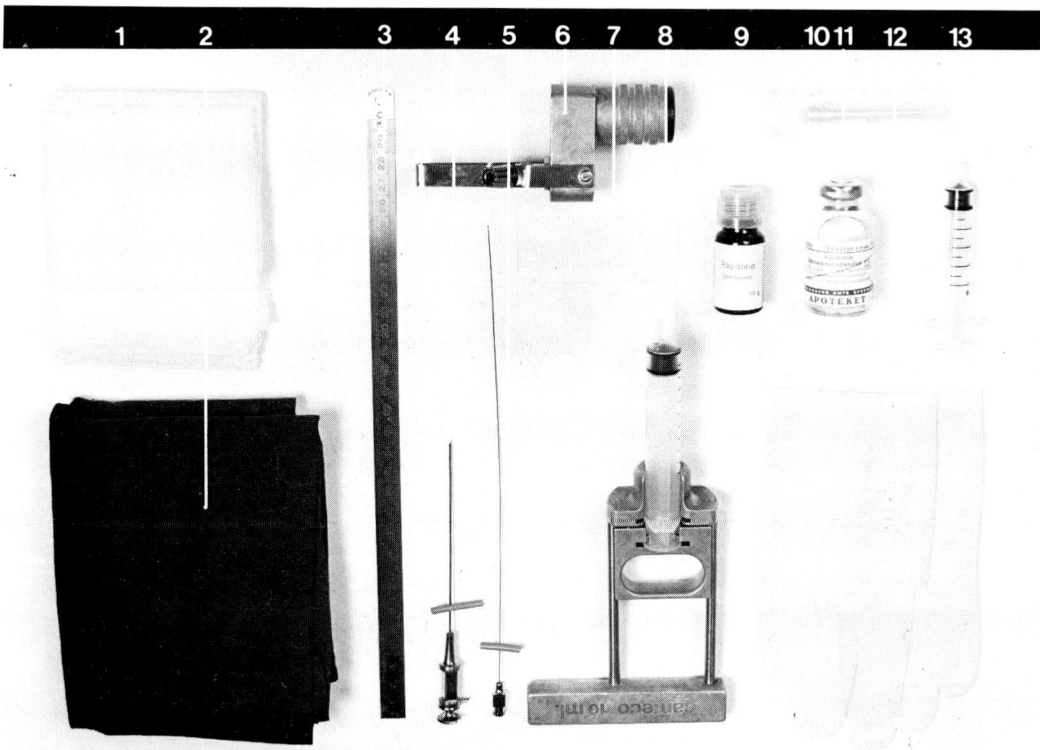

Fig. 5.1. *Equipment for fine needle aspiration biopsy*
1. Gauze swabs, 2. Sterile drape, 3. Ruler, 4. 19-gauge guide needle (outer diameter 1.2 mm) 5. 23-gauge biopsy needle (outer diameter 0.6 mm), 6. Biopsy transducer with a central canal, and connector placed off-axis, 7. Glass slides, 8. 10-ml syringe attached to aspiration handle (Camecon, Sweden), 9. Sterile oil, 10. Small needle for local anesthesia, 11. Local anesthetic (lidocain-noradrenaline 1%), 12. Gloves, 13. 5 ml-syringe for local anesthesia.

diameter 0.6 mm), a special aspiration handle and a 10-ml syringe (Fig. 5.1) the items necessary to perform the fine needle aspiration biopsy are exactly identical to those used for other puncture procedures under ultrasonic guidance. (See page 29).

## PATIENT PREPARATION AND POST-BIOPSY PRECAUTION

Because of its minimal discomfort, thin needle aspiration biopsy can be performed in almost all patients, even if they are in poor clinical condition. Children or patients who for some reason cannot cooperate can be examined and biopsied under general anesthesia.

In cases where the liver or the pancreas is to be biopsied, a simple screening for hemorrhagic disorders is made, and the patient should be fasting prior to the procedure.

Inpatients are returned to the ward immediately, outpatients are observed in the laboratory for 1–2 hours after the biopsy. After biopsy from the liver or when traversing the liver, the patient should be observed in the hospital for 24 hours.

## PROCEDURE

The position of the patient and the scanning plane are chosen so that the suspected tumor lesion and adjacent organs are well visualized. The puncture site, puncture direction and depth are determined. Whenever possible traversing the liver is avoided.

The selected site for puncture is marked on the skin, which is then prepared and draped as for any sterile procedure. Local anesthetic is administered to the skin and subcutaneous tissue, and sterile oil is applied.

The ordinary transducer is replaced by the biopsy transducer, and the scan is repeated through the mark on the skin. The transducer is angulated until the electronic marker visualized on the TV-monitor coincides with the desired needle pathway.

A 18-gauge needle (outer diameter 1.2 mm) is used as an outer guide needle through the skin and immediately underlying tissue, to ensure needle stability and to allow multiple passes of the fine needle into the tumor. The thickness of the skin plus the height of the transducer are marked off on

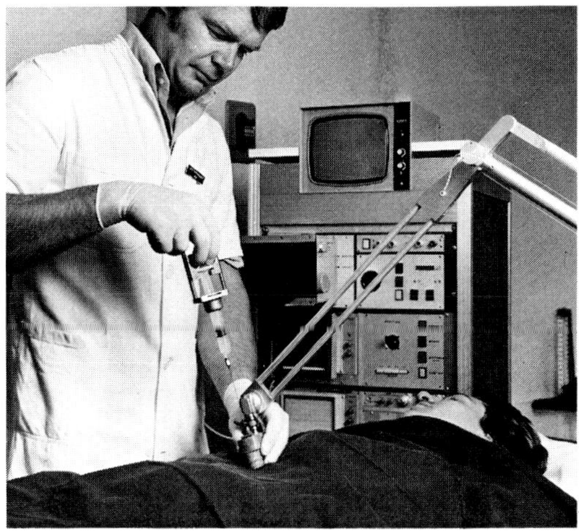

Fig. 5.2. *Fine needle aspiration biopsy*

the "guide needle" with a small piece of rubber to indicate needle stop. Another mark is placed on the thin needle, so this needle can reach into the center of the suspected mass when introduced through the guide needle.

The outer "guide needle" is now introduced via the transducer through the skin and subcutaneous tissue up to the mark. The fine needle fitted to a 10-ml syringe attached to a special aspiration handle (Fig. 5.2) is then introduced through the outer needle into the mass. The aspiration handle permits excellent single-hand manipulation.

When the tip of the fine needle is placed within the suspected tumor lesion, the aspiration handle is retracted completely, causing a vacuum in the syringe and the needle. The fine needle is moved back and forth in the tumor three or four times. The vacuum in the system is in most cases sufficient to obtain representative material for cytological examination.

When the aspiration is completed, it is mandatory that the negative pressure in the system be equilibrated before the needle is withdrawn, in order to prevent contamination of the aspirated material with cells from adjacent organs.

After withdrawal, the syringe is disconnected from the needle and filled with air, then reconnected, and the material in the needle is expelled onto a glass slide and smeared. (Fig. 5.3).

The fine needle biopsy may be repeated several times through the guide needle. The aspiration is made in various directions from the center of the mass and from the periphery, in order to obtain

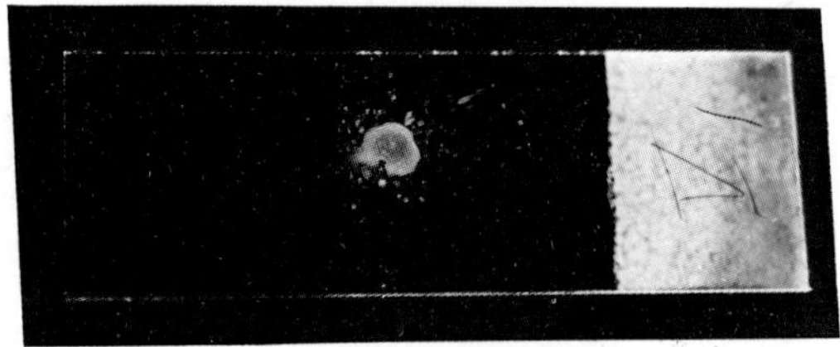

Fig. 5.3. *The aspirated material*
Before spread on the glass slide.

material from various parts of the tumor. Four or five passes with the fine needle are made routinely, and only a single drop of material is expelled on each glass slide.

With present, especially dynamic, equipment it is possible to visualize the needle or the needle tip during the insertion.

# References


Franzén, S., Giertz, G. and Zajicek, J.: Cytological diagnosis of prostatic tumours by transrectal biopsy – a preliminary report. *Br. J. Urol.* 32:193, 1960.

Holm, H. H., Kristensen, J. K., Rasmussen, S. N. Northeved, A. and Barlebo, H.: Ultrasound as a guide in percutaneous puncture technique. *Ultrasonics* 10:83, 1972.

Holm, H. H., Pedersen, J. F., Kristensen, J. K., Rasmussen, S. N., Hancke, S., and Jensen, F.: Ultrasonically guided percutaneous puncture. *Radiol. Clin. North Am.* 13:493, 1975.




Fine needle aspiration

# CHAPTER VI

# Aspiration biopsy cytology

Grete Krag Jacobsen

A close cooperation between the physician who performs the biopsy and the cytologist is of great importance. Together with the aspirated material relevant clinical information, in addition to information obtained during the biopsy procedure (location of the lesion, size, consistency, whether it is solid or cystic, etc.) must be given to the cytologist, because these variables have to be considered when the smear is evaluated.

However, the cytologist may be skillful and experienced, but if the technical quality of the smear is bad, he will not be able to give a satisfactory interpretation.

## Spreading of the aspirated material

Aspiration from a solid lesion is usually done in several different directions to yield representative material. The aspirated material is expelled in single droplets on glass slides, which have been properly cleaned for dust and greasy finger prints. The material is immediately spread using the edge of another glass slide, as for usual blood smears (Fig. 6.1). Tissue fragments are squeezed with the glass slide. One must take care to make a uniform thin-layered spread without jerking. This method is most suitable when the material is liquid or hemorrhagic. When the material is very rich in cells and without blood contamination, spreading between two ordinary glass slides using a flat pressure is better (Fig. 6.2). Usually 8 to 16 glass slides will be available for evaluation (Fig. 6.3). When large amounts of cyst fluid are obtained, the aspirate is centrifuged, placed on a glass slide and spread as described.

## Fixation and staining of the aspirated material

The specimen may be wet fixed or air dried. Wet fixation in 95% ethanol for at least 15 minutes is a widely used method, which is often followed by

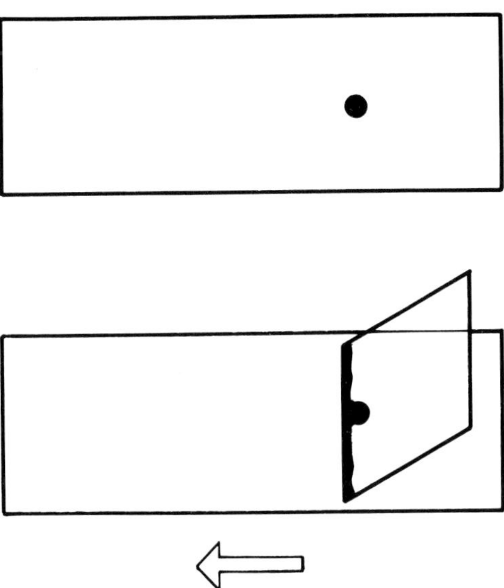

Fig. 6.1. *Smearing method 1.*
A small drop is placed on an ordinary rectangular clean glass slide. A cover glass of a counting chamber or a specially made large, thick glass is used for the spreading. At an angle of 45°, the spreading glass is placed in front of the drop to the left. Then it is moved to the right just to touch the drop which then runs along the edge of the spreading glass. Smearing is done evenly by moving the spreading glass to the left in one single movement.

staining according to the Papanicolaou technique. The wet fixation preserves nuclear details in an excellent way, so that optimal resemblance between the aspirated cells and the corresponding cells in the tissue is obtained. However, the method is sensitive to partial air drying before wet fixation, resulting in variability in fixation and nuclear staining properties. Air drying causes a minor loss of nuclear details, but these changes will be consistent in appearance from smear to smear. This method with "standardized artefacts" is prefered in many laboratories. The air-dried smears are stained according to the May-Grünwald-Giemsa technique, a staining which has been

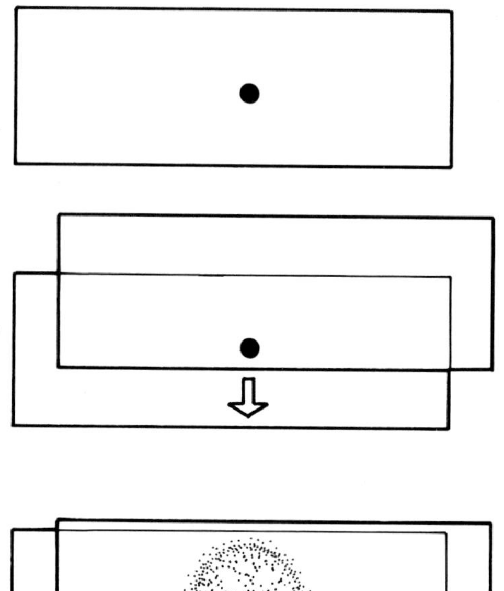

Fig. 6.2. *Smearing method 2.*
A small drop is expelled on an ordinary glass slide which has been carefully cleaned. Another glass slide of the same type is gently placed on top of the first one. The drop spreads immediately between the glasses which are drawn in opposite directions in a smooth movement. Both glasses are then available for further preparation and examination.

used for many years by hematologists for smears from blood and bone marrow. Cystic fluid is fixed and stained in the same way.

Smears for special cytochemical studies require special fixation that must be chosen before puncture, since once air dried, the smears cannot be refixated.

Finally it should be mentioned, that it is possible to fixate, stain and screen the smear within 30 minutes. During that time the patient may remain in the examination room and another biopsy may be obtained, if the first one does not yield sufficient material for conclusive diagnosis.

## Cytologic evaluation

At first the cytologist gets a general impression of the specimen regarding the quality, cellularity, distribution of cells or tissue fragments, and forms an estimate of the correlation between the information obtained about the nature of the lesion and the character of the specimen.

Fig. 6.3. *Examples of bad and good films.*
1. The drop was too big, and the spreading was unevenly done. The glass slide was left on a slanting support which made the material run backwards.
2. Only half of the glass is used and part of the material is at the edge of the glass and not available for examination.
3. On the glass too much material with heavy blood contamination was expelled, making a thick, impenetrable film.
4 and 5. Two glass slides with the right amount of material spread in thin films, very suitable for microscopical examination.

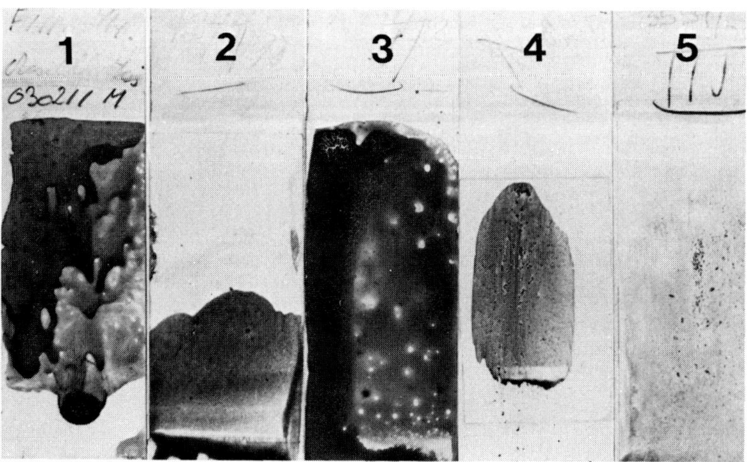

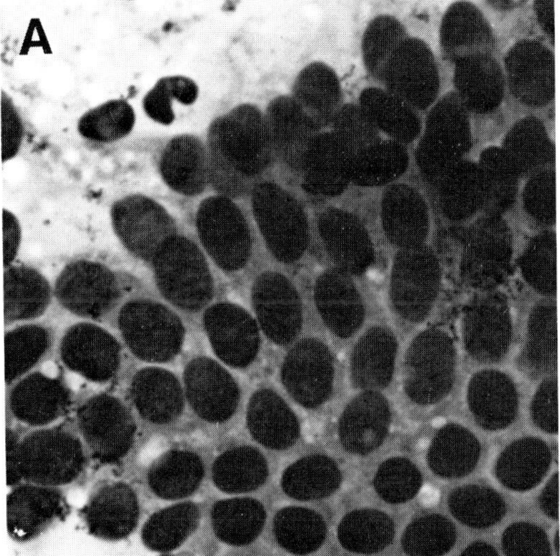

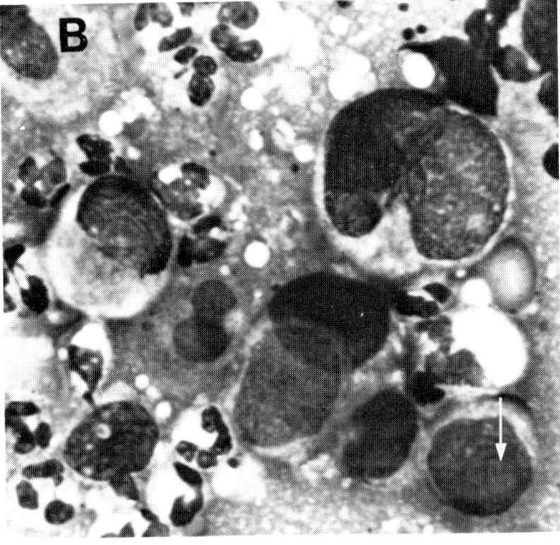

Fig. 6.4. *Aspiration biopsies demonstrating normal cells and cancer cells from the pancreas.*
A. Normal ductular cells in a regular pattern with a good cohesion between the cells are seen. B. Tumor cells are present singly or in small clusters on a necrotic background. The tumor cells are pleomorphic with macronucleoli (arrow-marked) and hypercromatic nuclei, some of which are multiple. × 400.

The details are then studied. It must be emphasized that the aspirate consists of a cellular material and on a background. Recognition of malignant cells is based on well-known cytologic criteria of malignancy. Briefly, these criteria are based on nuclear characteristics, i.e. enlargement of nuclei with increase of nucleo-cytoplasmic ratio, variation in size, and shape (pleomorphism) and structure, in addition to hyperchromasia, macronucleoli and mitoses (Fig. 6.4).

The presence of two or more of these characteristics is necessary for identifying a cell as a malignant cell. The interpretation of malignancy will be more reliable if the changes are found in many cells, although a few cells with outspoken alterations may suffice for a correct diagnosis of malignancy.

An evaluation of the arrangement of the cells is of great importance, too. Normal cells with normal intercellular cohesion are arranged in single-layer sheets with a regular pattern, whereas tumor cells often are present in thick clusters or as single cells.

The background of the smear on which the cells are present may give information of considerable importance. Observation of blood, inflammatory cells, microorganisms, secreted material, necrotic cells or tissue fragments in varying amounts and mixtures is of extreme value in obtaining a correct diagnosis.

To obtain maximum accuracy of the method, one has to be aware of its limitations. For example, not all malignant cells fulfill the usual cytologic criteria of malignancy and may therefore cause insoluble diagnostic problems. Inflammation and regeneration may produce changes which resemble some of the nuclear characteristics of the malignant cell.

Besides being subject to misinterpretation, any biopsy is subject to sampling error. For example, some tumors may be surrounded by or contain fibrous tissue, and aspiration from such an area will not produce tumor cells.

Finally, it should be stressed that the absence of tumor cells in an aspiration biopsy is of limited value and by itself never excludes the presence of a malignant lesion.

# References

Esposti, P. L., Franzén, S. and Zajicek, J.: The aspiration biopsy smear. In: L. G. Koss: Diagnostic Cytology and its Histopathologic Basis. 2nd Edition, *J. B. Lippincott,* Philadelphia, 1968.

Söderström, N.: Fine Needle Aspiration Biopsy: Used as a Direct Adjunct in Clinical Diagnostic Work. *Almqvist and Wiksell,* Stockholm, 1966.

Zajicek, J.: Aspiration Biopsy Cytologi, Part I. Cytology of Supradiaphragmatic Organs. Vol. 4, Monographs in Clinical Cytology. *S. Karper,* Basel, 1974.

# CHAPTER VII

# Bacteriology

Tage Justesen

Ultrasonically guided needle aspiration is a refined method for obtaining material for bacteriological examination. The precise location of the needle will ensure that relevant material is aspirated and local instillation of antibiotics can be performed after aspiration. In certain situations this procedure seems to be curative so that surgical intervention can be avoided (see chapter XVI). The aspiration procedure by itself does not seem to represent any danger concerning further infectious spread (see chapter IV).

## THE NORMAL MICROBIAL FLORA AND INFECTION

The skin and mucous membranes always harbor a variety of microorganisms, some of which are potentially pathogenic. These organisms are adapted to the non-invasive mode of life, but if removed from their natural environment and introduced into the tissues these organisms may become pathogenic.

The highest concentration of bacteria is normally found in the large bowel. Stools represent a 25% suspension of viable bacteria of which 99.9% are anaerobic. Thus spillage of colonic content, whether due to trauma, diverticulitis or appendicitis, inflammatory bowel disease, carcinoma or surgery, is associated with a high incidence of especially anaerobic intra-abdominal infections. When an abscess results, it may occur within the peritoneal cavity, retroperitoneally or intraparenchymally. The vast majority of these infections are associated with one or more anaerobes and aerobes. Virtually all of these usually polymicrobial infections yield *Bacteroides fragilis, Clostridium spp., Peptostreptococcus spp.* or *Peptococcus spp.* as well as *E. coli* or other enterobactericeae, enterococci and Pseudomonas.

The normal flora in the mouth and vagina also contains a considerable amount of potentially pathogenic anaerobic bacteria. It is well known that abscess formation in the lungs is often due to bacteria derived from the oral cavity which is probably also the case in brain abscesses. A similar role is played by anaerobic bacteria when infections originate in relation to the female genital tract.

The demonstration of a single known pathogen does not leave many problems but the types of infections described here are typical examples of synergistic bacterial interaction and the recovery of a mixture of anaerobic and aerobic bacteria has often left the clinician with the impression that the whole thing was insignificant. Up till now it is still difficult to point out the specific pathogenic organism in such mixtures but it should be stressed that anaerobic bacteria, especially *B. fragilis,* are often found in *pure* culture as the single causative organism.

## PRINCIPLES FOR BACTERIOLOGICAL EXAMINATION

Several problems must be solved to ensure relevant bacteriological examination. The bacteriological sample consists of more than just a side remark to the nurse about also remembering to send something to the microbiologist.

In the present context some of the major problems follow below.

## Information

In the first place it is important to stress that the clinician will obtain maximum information from the microbiologist by indicating the sampling procedure, the sampling location and a qualified judgment of the nature and origin of the infection. This will enable the microbiologist to perform examinations not covered by "routine procedures", i.e. staining for acid-fast bacteria, quantitation of bacteria, use of selective media and anaerobic cultivation.

## Contamination

In cases where material is obtained by needle aspiration, the needle has to be introduced through the skin or through a mucous membrane. The normal skin flora consists mainly of *Staphylococcus epidermidis* and the anaerobic nonspore-forming Gram-positive rod *Propionibacterium acnes*. Contamination of bacteriological specimens with these two organisms is a well-known phenomenon in blood cultivation systems due to incomplete disinfection of the skin. Since these organisms from time to time can act as pathogenic bacteria, any confusion should be avoided using proper skin disinfection. Even if samples are contaminated with skin bacteria a quantitative culture technique will compensate for misinterpretations since only small amounts of the organisms will be present. Therefore it is not recommended to use blood sampling equipment for collection and transportation of aspirated samples.

## Aspiration

Aspirated material should be obtained in a sterile syringe without addition of any kind. The minimum amount of material for a thorough bacteriological examination is about 2 ml. If this amount is not available it is recommended to soak a carbon impregnated swab and place it in Stuarts transport medium or a similar transport medium. Blood culture systems and dry swabs should be avoided. It should be pointed out that swabs are unsuited for the preparation of microscopic slides.

## Transportation

The result of a bacteriological examination is highly dependent on proper transportation of the specimens. On one hand no multiplication should occur with resulting overgrowth of certain less fastidious microorganisms, and on the other survival of fastidious bacteria should be ensured together with the maintenance of the original mutual proportions between the bacterial species. These demands can be met to a great extent by reducing the transportation period to the least possible, i.e. within 1 hour. Means for proper transportation include

1) Syringe technique, i.e. elimination of all air from the specimen-containing syringe and needle, and sticking the needle into a sterile rubber stopper.

2) Injection of the specimen into a sterile, oxygen-free glass tube containing $CO_2$ or $N_2$.

Alternatively, a tube can be flushed with $CO_2$ or $N_2$ to evacuate atmospheric air and then stoppered immediately after the injection of the specimen. If the transportation time is short, method 1) is sufficient, but if transportation is delayed method 2) is recommended. If swabs have to be used (only in an emergency) the specimen should be preserved in Stuarts transport medium or in a similar commercially available transport system. The specimen should be kept at ambient temperature when transportation time is short but kept at 4°C if transportation is delayed.

It should be stressed that the described procedures also facilitate the survival of aerobic growing organisms.

## Cultivation

Cultivation should be performed anaerobically as well as aerobically. For the anaerobic cultivation a reliable technique should be used. An evacuation replacement jar, "Gas pack" or "Gas kit" type of jars, roll tubes or anaerobic chambers are satisfactory, provided that active catalysts are used together with an atmosphere containing at least 3% $H_2$.

Quantitative cultivation should be done aerobically as well as anaerobically to help exclude contaminants and to determine the prevalent organism.

Antibiotic sensitivity testing should be done for all isolated pathogens for the purpose of rational antibiotic treatment.

*B. fragilis* is the anaerobic bacteria most often isolated from intraabdominal abscesses and it should be noted that this organism is highly resistant to aminoglucosides and penicillins but almost invariably sensitive to metronidazole and clindamycin.

## References


Drasar, B. S. and Hill, M. J.: Human intestinal flora. *Academic Press,* London, New York, San Francisco, 1974.

Finegold, S. M.: Anaerobic bacteria in human disease. *Academic Press Inc.,* New York, 1977.

# CHAPTER VIII

# Ultrasonically guided puncture of renal mass lesions

Jørgen Kvist Kristensen and Grete Krag Jacobsen

The ultrasonic diagnosis of a renal mass lesion and its differentiation into solid or cystic are usually very reliable. In a typical case of solid renal tumor it is seen to break the contour of the kidney and to displace the sinus echoes. It is irregularly outlined and internal echoes indicate its solid nature (Fig. 8.1).

A typical renal cyst also breaks the contour of the kidney and displaces the sinus echoes. It has sharply delineated walls and a completely echo-free interior. Behind the cyst echo enhancement is usually observed (Fig. 8.2). However, further diagnostic information may be obtained by supplementary use of ultrasonically guided puncture.

## PUNCTURE TECHNIQUE

When a renal mass lesion has been demonstrated ultrasonically and a percutaneous puncture is to be performed, the optimum site and direction for the introduction of the needle have to be considered. Although a diagnosis of a renal mass lesion, at least of the right kidney, can frequently be obtained with the patient in the supine position, it may be advisable to confirm the diagnosis with prone scans, and for the puncture it *is* advisable to perform it with the patient prone, possibly in the lateral decubitus position. When possible, the needle should be inserted caudal to the ribs. Intercostal scanning may give contact problems and slight displacement of the transducer causes rib shadowing. In addition, with subcostal insertion of the needle, puncture of the pleura is avoided. Laterally the bowel can usually be identified and it is preferable in cases of anteriorly located renal mass lesions to pass a fine needle through renal tissue rather than through bowel. With these reservations in mind, the attempt to insert the needle through the posterior abdominal wall directly into the mass may be made.

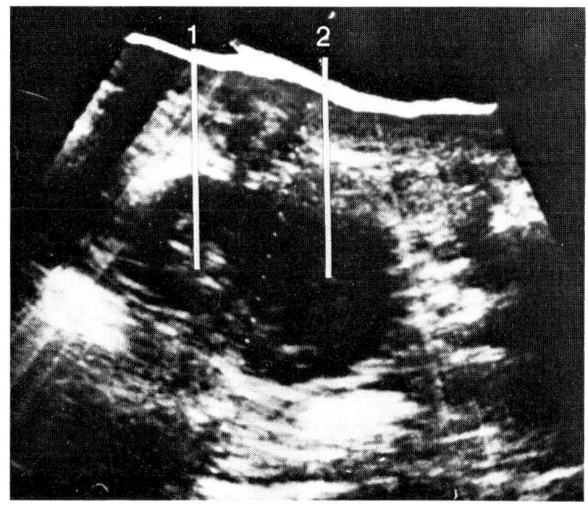

Fig. 8.1. *Solid renal tumor scan*
Longitudinal scan through left kidney, prone position. 1. Normal cranial part of kidney, 2. Solid mass in caudal part.

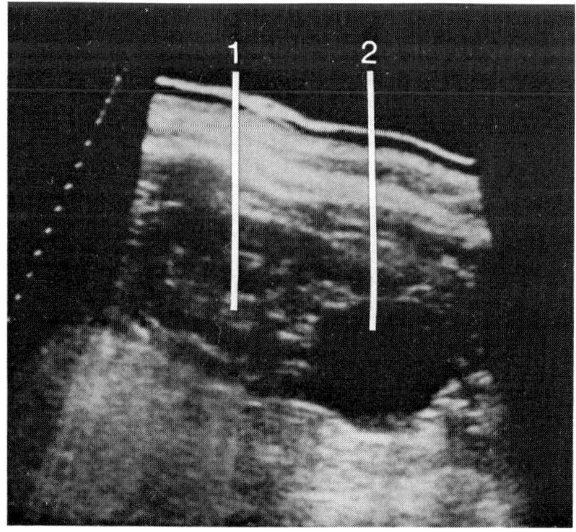

Fig. 8.2. *Renal cyst scan*
Longitudinal scan through right kidney, prone position. 1. Normal cranial part of kidney, 2. Cyst in caudal part.

The puncture site and direction are chosen with the patient in shallow respiration, in case of small lesions, possibly in apnoea. If access to a mass is difficult because of overlying ribs, deep inspiration may facilitate the puncture by bringing the mass into an intercostal space or distal to the ribs. Occasionally it is advantageous to place a pillow under the abdomen of the patient. Scans may be improved with this and it has a tendency to diminish the respiratory excursions of the kidney.

Renal mass lesions should almost invariably be punctured through the puncture transducer. When a cyst has been diagnosed from the scans, a 1.2 mm needle is chosen, whereas a solid lesion should be punctured with a 0.6 mm fine needle inserted via a 1.2 mm guide needle. If the scans do not allow a satisfactory differentiation between cystic and solid, it is advisable to use the fine needle for puncture. If fluid is aspirated, the fine needle is removed and the guide needle introduced into the lesion for easier aspiration. In case of a mass lesion in the renal hilum the fine needle should be used because of the possibility of traversing the large vessels centrally in the kidney.

## INVESTIGATIONS IN RELATION TO PUNCTURE OF CYSTIC LESIONS

The fluid of a simple kidney cyst is usually clear, and yellowish. During aspiration it may turn slightly red due to needle trauma of the cyst wall. Some cysts contain chocolate-colored fluid due to previous hemorrhage. In some cases the fluid may be opaque because of a high protein content, and in case of an infected cyst the aspirate may be puslike.

Quantitative emptying of a punctured kidney cyst should be attempted in order to test the aspirated volume in relation to the estimated volume of the mass. The volume of a mass seen on the scans is calculated from the formula of a sphere $(4/3 \times \pi \times r^3)$, r being the radius of the mass). Aspiration should give at least 75% of this volume in order that it can be considered a quantitative emptying. The figure 75% has been set arbitrarily. If quantitative emptying is not possible, it may indicate that a multicystic lesion was punctured, or a cystic area within a solid lesion. Also the possibility exists that the renal pelvis is inadvertently punctured and the fluid withdrawn is actually urine. With small peripelvic masses this may very well happen.

The biochemical composition of cyst fluid has been investigated in an effort to elucidate the etiology of kidney cyst formation and to find parameters indicating or excluding malignancy. The electrolyte concentration of cyst fluid is identical to that of plasma, as is the concentration of creatinine, whereas the concentration of urea and glucose tends to be slightly elevated. The protein content of cyst fluid varies a great deal, but in uncomplicated cases it is always smaller than in plasma, whereas in cases of infection it is greatly elevated. Usually there are no lipids present in a cyst and if so, this has been used as an indicator of malignancy. This test seems to be rather sensitive, but not very specific. The lactic dehydrogenase content of cyst fluid is very low but has been reported to be elevated in cases of malignancy.

The differentiation between cyst fluid and urine is easily accomplished by the examination of the aspirated fluid and a urine specimen with a lab stick, because usually there is neither glucose nor protein in the urine. If this should be the case, creatinine concentrations can be used for differentiation.

Cytologic examination of the fluid should be routine. From the cytologist's point of view, as much fluid should be aspirated as possible in order to provide as much cellular material as possible. Usually the fluid from a simple kidney cyst contains no or few cells. Some of these may be of epithelial origin, being desquamated from the inside of the cyst wall. Even when partly disintegrated they will in most cases cause no diagnostic problems. The cell background of the centrifuged, smeared cyst fluid is most often clean, but sometimes protein precipitations are present. Erythrocytes in varying amounts may be encountered due to needle trauma of the cyst wall. With inflammatory reactions, leucocytes will be present, possibly intermingled with debris in the case of pus formation.

Injection of a contrast medium into kidney cysts for subsequent radiographic delineation can also be accomplished when the puncture is performed under ultrasound guidance. Usually the cyst is partially aspirated and the aspirated volume replaced by a water-soluble contrast medium, or the cyst is emptied completely with subsequent replacement by one-third water-soluble contrast medium and two-thirds carbon dioxide. Such single or double contrast studies are considered very important by some, too laborious by others.

If the cyst is not totally expanded to original volume, wall irregularities may be demonstrated on the radiograms with a subsequent erroneous diagnosis of tumor growth in the wall. If too large a volume is injected, the cyst may rupture. The addition of a third, oily contrast agent, usually panthopaque, has also been advocated for the purpose of preventing recurrence of the cyst because of the sclerosing effect of the medium. Also the value of this procedure is debatable. Even simple aspiration of cysts will cause shrinkage or disappearance in a number of cases, but this rate is probably higher with the injection of panthopaque. However, this may produce a severe, localized inflammatory reaction, resulting in pain and a rise in temperature. The problem with kidney cysts is in most cases only a diagnostic one, and only on rare occasions is there a need for therapy, e.g. when a large cyst causes pain or when a cyst causes calyceal obstruction. In the latter cases it may be worthwhile to try the possible effect of panthopaque.

## INVESTIGATIONS IN RELATION TO PUNCTURE OF SOLID LESIONS

The macroscopic evaluation of the fine needle aspirate from a solid lesion is difficult. The idea is to fill only the needle with cellular material. Expelled and smeared on glass slides, such a proper aspirate is usually seen to be slightly bloody with small tissue particles. This may, however, also be the appearance of an aspirate from normal renal tissue. If bloody material comes into the syringe, it may indicate the puncture of a blood vessel or a tumor area with hemorrhage. If unclear, white-yellowish fluid is aspirated, it may indicate the puncture of a necrotic tumor area or possibly a tuberculous abscess. In such cases the aspiration should be repeated from other areas of the lesion as well as if no material is obtained. To have an immediate microscopic evaluation of the aspirate may save the patient another visit to the ultrasound laboratory. With a good collaboration with the cytologist, air drying, fixation and staining may be accomplished in 20 minutes and a quick microscopic survey will reveal if the aspiration should be repeated.

The cytologist should be provided with relevant information when the specimen is sent to him. He should be told if the punctured lesion most likely is a hypernephroma or a transitional cell tumor, or if there is a likehood that the lesion may be metastatic. It is also important to indicate the location of the lesion, because a cytologic specimen from the adrenal may be confused with a specimen from a clear cell hypernephroma. If the lesion is located caudally in the kidney, concern about such a possible diagnostic error is avoided. The chance that a tuberculous lesion has been punctured should also be stated so that the cytologist can take precautions against spread of infectious material and apply proper staining.

On the final cytologic evaluation normal kidney cells may be present either solely or together with tumor cells. In aspirates from normal parts of a kidney, epithelial cells are found in most varying amounts and their appearance may also vary according to the parts of the nephrons that have been hit (Fig. 8.3). Endothelial cells and stroma cells may be encountered and if a calyx or the renal pelvis has been punctured, urothelial cells may be seen.

*Renal adenomas* will produce aspirates of varying cellularity, ranging from that which can be obtained from the normal parenchyma or from the highly cellular carcinoma. The cells are usually rather uniform epithelial cells with almost normal

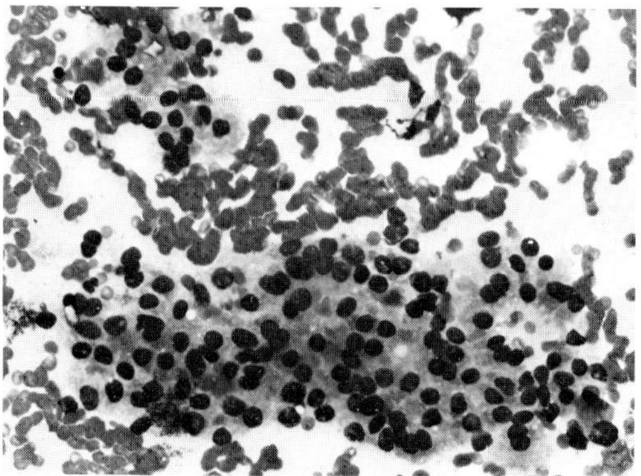

Fig. 8.3. *Normal kidney cytology*
Uniform tubular epithelial cells in regular arrangement are seen on a blood contaminated but otherwise clean background without inflammatory cells or necrotic debris.

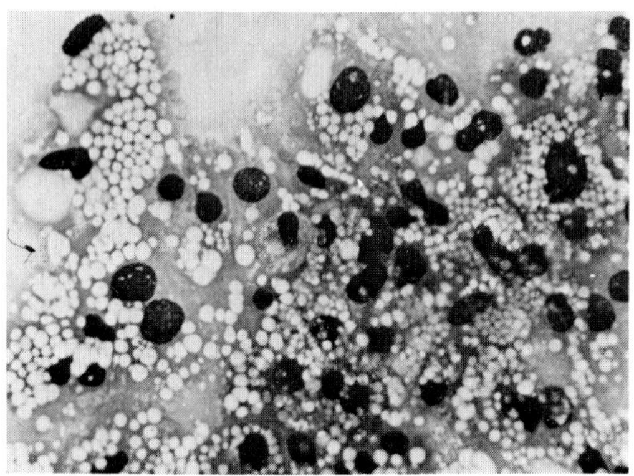

Fig. 8.4. *Renal clear cell carcinoma cytology*
Irregular sheets of cells with abundant, highly vacuolated cytoplasm and moderately pleomorphic nuclei are characteristic of this tumor type.

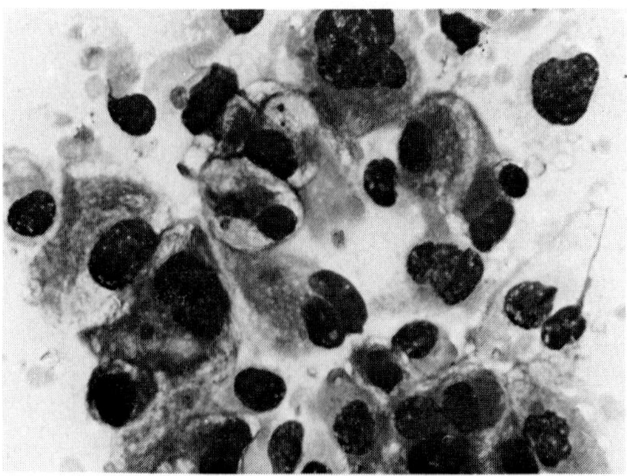

Fig. 8.5. *Low differentiated renal carcinoma cytology*
Epithelial cells in clusters, irregularly arranged are present. The cells and nuclei are pleomorphic, accumulation of chromatin in the nucleus results in hyperchromasia and the nucleus/cytoplasm ratio is increased. In many cases such poorly differentiated carcinomas have lost completely cytologic characteristics of origin from the renal parenchyma or urothelium.

appearance or with only subtle changes. Such a microscopic picture may be difficult or even impossible to differentiate cytologically into a renal adenoma or a well-differentiated carcinoma. Even histologically this differentiation may be impossible.

*Renal carcinomas* (hypernephromas) which form the vast majority of renal tumors usually have an easily diagnosable cytologic appearance (Figs 8.4 and 8.5). The cellularity is usually very high. The main type of cells encountered are clear cells with a pale, vacuolated, abundant cytoplasm and relatively small, slightly pleomorphic and somewhat pycnotic nuclei, and granular cells which contain a finely granular cytoplasm. In some tumors only one type of cells is present while others are of mixed composition. Also the shape and size of cells and nuclei vary from one tumor to another, denoting the degree of differentiation and also within the same tumor varying differentiation may be observed. This makes it important to obtain aspirates from various parts of a tumor. Also because some renal adenocarcinomas contain areas with sarcomatoid differentiation it is important to obtain aspirates from more than one direction in order that the true nature of the lesion can be disclosed.

*Tumors which originate from the urothelium* of the renal pelvis or the calyces usually yield very cellular aspirates with epithelial cells in papillary formations (Fig. 8.6). With only slight or moderate variations in size and shape of cells and nuclei,

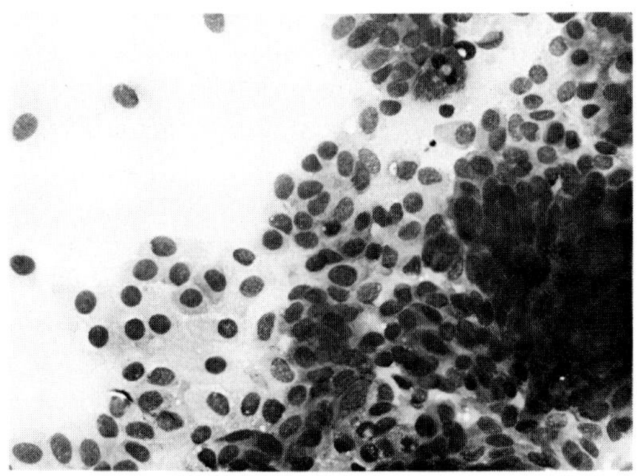

Fig. 8.6. *Urothelial cell carcinoma cytology*
Fairly uniform epithelial cells with slightly enlarged nuclei and finely granular cytoplasm are seen in sheets and small clusters of papillary configuration. The cytologic picture which still retains resemblance to urothelium is characteristic of a well-differentiated carcinoma of the renal pelvis or calyces.

the urothelial origin of the tumor may be fairly easily diagnosed, but with poorly differentiated tumors the cellular picture may be indistinguishable from that of poorly differentiated renal carcinomas or even other epithelial tumors.

*Other types of renal tumors,* primary such as benign or malignant mesenchymal tumors or secondary such as lymphomas, invasion from neighboring organs or metastases are rare but should be borne in mind when the cytologic picture is not characteristic of a renal carcinoma or urothelial cell carcinoma.

## RESULTS

When considering the results of ultrasonically guided puncture of renal mass lesions, the first problem is, with what accuracy a mass lesion can be punctured.

This was evaluated in a personal series of patients with cysts. Fluid was aspirated from 98 of 108 cysts giving a success rate of a little over 90%. This was in a consecutive series from the first 5 years of our experience with ultrasonically guided puncture and it included cysts down to 2 cm. With our present experience the accuracy is probably better.

The accuracy in hitting solid lesions is likely to be of the same order, but it can not be evaluated in the same way, because a solid aspirate does not necessarily mean that the lesion was hit and a nonmalignant cytologic diagnosis carries a false negative rate of its own.

The diagnostic accuracy of ultrasonically guided puncture of renal mass lesions combined with cytologic studies of the aspirate was evaluated in a consecutive series of 291 patients with suspected or known renal mass lesions.

Based upon strict criteria, a final diagnosis was obtained in 252 patients. All cytologic diagnoses were routine diagnoses reported to the clinical departments. From 105 patients fluid was aspirated (Table 8.I). There was one false positive diagnosis, a 2-cm cyst from which quantitative amounts of clear fluid were aspirated, containing cells which were suspected to originate from a well-differentiated hypernephroma. There was one false negative cytologic diagnosis, a 4-cm lesion of indeterminate structure on the scans. Quantitative amounts of brownish fluid without tumor cells were aspirated. The patient turned out to have renal metastases with hemorrhage and necrosis from a pulmonary carcinoma. There was one malignant cyst which appeared as a large, simple cyst in all respects except for tumor cells in the aspirate. Histological sections showed the inner surface of its wall covered with small papillary formations of epithelial tumor tissue. The three cases of malignant tumors with fluid aspirates were all solid on the scans and only small quantities of unclear fluid could be withdrawn.

Using the following criteria for a cyst:
1) typical cyst on the scans
2) quantitative emptying
3) no tumor cells in the aspirate,
there were no malignancies misdiagnosed.

In the same series there were 149 patients with a solid aspirate (Table 8.II). It is not possible to tell how many of the 17 malignant tumors without tumor cells in the aspirate were not hit and how many were cytologically false negatives. This series is also consecutively representing our experience from the first 7 years of ultrasonically guided renal puncture. A primary cytologic evaluation of the aspirate and possible repuncture would propably have reduced the number of cases without tumor cells and the number of indeterminate ones. The 10 simple cysts were definitely not hit. Aspirates from one simple cyst, two non-

Table 8.1. *105 Patients with fluid aspirate*

| Final diagnosis | Cytology | +Tumor cells | −Tumor cells | Indeterminate |
|---|---|---|---|---|
| Simple cyst | | 1 | 95 | 2 |
| Malignant cyst | | 1 | − | − |
| Malignant tumor | | 3 | 1 | − |
| Hydro-pyonephrosis | | − | − | 2 |

Table 8.2. *149 Patients with solid aspirate*

| Final diagnosis | Cytology | +Tumor cells | −Tumor cells | Indeterminate |
|---|---|---|---|---|
| Malignant tumor | | 103 | 17 | 4 |
| Simple cyst | | 1 | 8 | 1 |
| Miscellaneous disorders | | 2 | 3 | − |
| Normal kidney | | 2 | 8 | − |

malignant disorders and two normal kidneys were considered to contain tumor cells. The two non-malignant disorders represented unspecific inflammation and tuberculosis, respectively. Possible explanations for the false positive cytological diagnoses in the cyst case and the two normal kidneys are: misdiagnosis because of the numerous types of cells present in the normal kidney (cf. p. 8.9), aspirate from an otherwise undetected, small cortical adenoma, inadvertent puncture of the adrenal gland.

Although cytology carries false positives and false negatives, it is very reliable in the diagnosis of simple cysts and it may be helpful in the evaluation of solid lesions.

## COMPLICATIONS

Complications were registered only in one patient in the above-mentioned series. One patient with a solid tumor was found to have a large perirenal hematoma at surgery 5 days after puncture.

In a survey of complications in renal cyst puncture and aspiration, the complication rate in almost 2000 punctures performed in institutions with extensive experience was 1.1% major complications. The vast majority of complications were perirenal hemorrhage and pneumothorax. The clinical significance of these complications was not stated, but even a complication rate of approximately 1% compares favorably with that in a series of 150 surgical explorations for renal cysts with only 52% uneventful recoveries. Also the fact that the ultrasonically guided puncture can be performed on an outpatient basis compares favorably to the hospital stay after surgical exploration.

## INDICATIONS

The use of ultrasonically guided percutaneous puncture of renal mass lesions is suggested in the following situations:

1) All lesions appearing on the scans as cysts should be punctured for final diagnosis – and treatment in the sense that no treatment is required of a simple cyst unless its size and location may cause local symptoms

2) Arteriographically avascular lesions, because 5% of solid lesions appear avascular on arteriography

3) When radiologic investigations of an ultrasonically solid lesion are indeterminate

4) When arteriography of an ultrasonically solid lesion is contra-indicated, for instance in allergy to contrast media

5) In suspected abscesses which can be diagnosed and treated with puncture as described in chapter XVI.

## References


Becker, J. A. and Schneider, M.: Simple cyst of the kidney. *Sem. Roentgenol.* 10:103, 1975.

Beyer, D. and Fiedler, V.: Ist die Nierenzystenpunktion eine brauchbare Methode zur Differentialdiagnostik gefässarmer raumfordernder Nierenprozesse. *Urologe A* 16:339, 1977.

Kristensen, J. K., Holm, H. H., Rasmussen, S. N. and Barlebo, H.: Ultrasonically guided percutaneous puncture of renal masses. *Scand. J. Urol. Nephrol.* 6, suppl. 15:49, 1972.

Lang, E. K., Johnson, B., Chance, H. L., Enright, J. R., Fontenot, R., Trichel, B. E., Wood, M., Brown, R. and Martin, E. C. St.: Assessment of avascular renal mass lesions. *South. Med. J.* 65:1, 1972.

Lang, E. K.: Renal cyst puncture and aspiration: A survey of complications. *Am. J. Roentgenol.* 128:723, 1977.

Pollack, H. M., Goldberg, B. B., Morales, J. O. and Bogash, M.: Systematized approach to the differential diagnosis of renal masses. *Radiology* 113:653, 1974.

Stanisic, T. H. and Grayhack, J. T.: Morbidity and mortality of renal exploration for cyst. *Surg. Gynecol. Obstet.* 145:733, 1977.

Steg, A.: Renal cysts. Chemical and dynamic study of cystic fluid. *Eur. Urol.* 2:164, 1976.

Steg, A.: Renal cysts in adults. Clinical aspect and diagnostical approach based on the analysis of 1342 cases. *Eur. Urol.* 2:209, 1976.

Vestby, G. W.: Perkutane Behandlung von Nierenzysten. *Acta Radiol.* 11:529, 1971.

Wettlaufer, J. N. and Modarelli, R. O.: Tripple contrast percutaneous nephrocystography and analysis of cyst aspirate. *Urol.* 12:373, 1978.

Zajicek, J.: Aspiration cytology biopsy. Part 2: Cytology of Infradiaphragmatic Organs. Vol. 4, Monographs in Clinical Cytology. *S. Karger,* Basel, 1979.

# CHAPTER IX

# Ultrasonically guided nephrostomy

Jan Fog Pedersen

Patients with acute post-renal uremia in whom retrograde passage of catheters into the ureters is impossible present a difficult clinical problem. Emergency surgery with diverting nephrostomy has previously been necessary, but involves considerable operative risk.

Percutaneous nephrostomy under fluoroscopic guidance for both diagnostic and therapeutic purposes has been performed for several years. Obviously, a prerequisite for successful percutaneous puncture is adequate visualization of the dilated renal pelvis. This is often impossible urographically with uremic patients or results in considerable delay in treatment of those patients with slow but persistent renal excretion of contrast material.

In contrast, the ultrasonic visualization of the kidney is independent of renal function, so it is possible in the uremic or anuric patient to diagnose obstructive hydronephrosis with a dilated renal pelvis and to puncture it under ultrasonic guidance (Fig. 9.1).

## Method

With the patient in the prone position the optimum site for puncture is defined and marked on the skin. This should be as far laterally as possible in order to reduce discomfort and catheter kinking

when the patient lies on his back. In order not to puncture the colon or the peritoneum, the direction of puncture should have an angle to the sagital plane of no more than 45°. The lateral introduction of the catheter – to avoid catheter kinking – means that the needle will traverse the renal parenchyma before it enters the renal pelvis. Thereby the risk of puncturing hilar vessels is re-

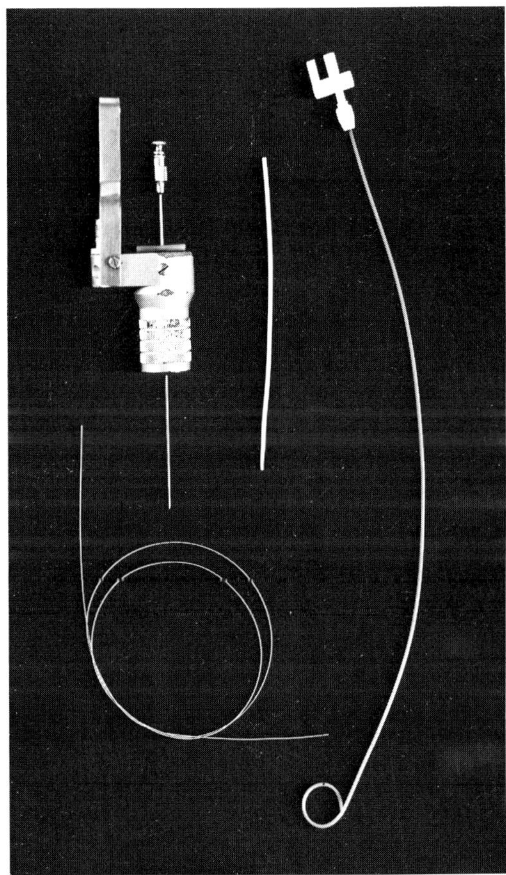

Fig. 9.2. *Equipment for ultrasonically guided nephrostomy*
Top left, puncture transducer with 1.2 mm lumbar needle inserted. In the middle, short, stiff 2.0 mm dilating catheter. Right, 1.9 mm soft polyethylene catheter with curved, multiholed tip. Bottom, guide wire.

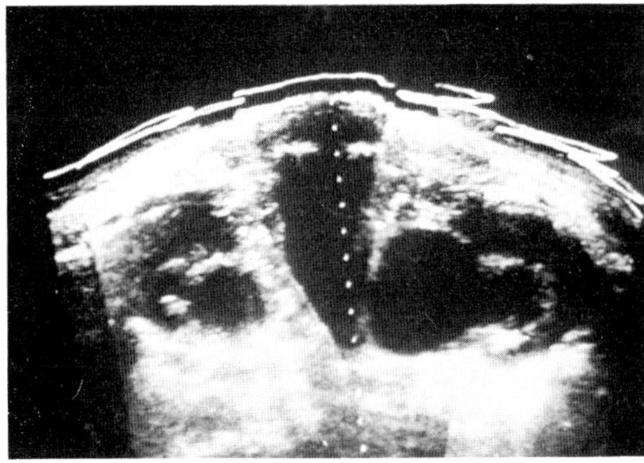

Fig. 9.1. *Bilateral hydronephrosis*
Transverse scan, prone position. 1. 2×3 cm dilated pelvis of left kidney, 2. 4×6 cm dilated pelvis of right kidney.

duced, especially if the pelvis is punctured as far caudally in the kidney as possible.

Local anesthetic is applied, the skin is swabbed with iodine, smeared with sterile contact medium and the scan is reproduced with the sterilized puncture transducer (Fig. 9.2). While the transducer is directed toward the renal pelvis a lumbar needle, outer diameter 1.2 mm, is introduced through the transducer and inserted in the correct direction governed by the transducer into a depth already determined from the A-scope or the scan. (Fig. 9.3). The placement of the needle is assured from the appearance on the A-scope of the needle tip echo within the echo-free renal pelvis. Further confirmation is obtained when the stiletto is removed and urine emerges.

A soft-tipped 0.6 mm guide wire is then introduced through the needle well into the renal pelvis and the needle-transducer assembly is removed. Next a short, stiff catheter, 2.0 mm outer diameter, is inserted over the guide wire to dilate the puncture canal and removed. Finally, a 40 cm long, 1.9 mm outer diameter soft polyethylene catheter with a preshaped curve and four sideholes at the tip is introduced over the guide wire into the renal pelvis where it coils. The guide wire is removed and the catheter secured with a skin suture. Antegrade pyolography is performed when indicated (Fig. 9.4).

## Results

The procedure soon proved simple and benign in the uremic patients for whom it had been designed. Therefore the criteria for selection were expanded to also include patients with post-renal obstruction where excretory urography was unsatisfactory, and retrograde pyelography impossible, and patients with infected hydronephrosis causing fever and sepsis. With a transplanted kidney the procedure is identical but technically easier because of the superficial location of the graft.

Fourty-four nephrostomies were attempted. Thirty-six of the procedures were successful although six times the catheter slipped out of the

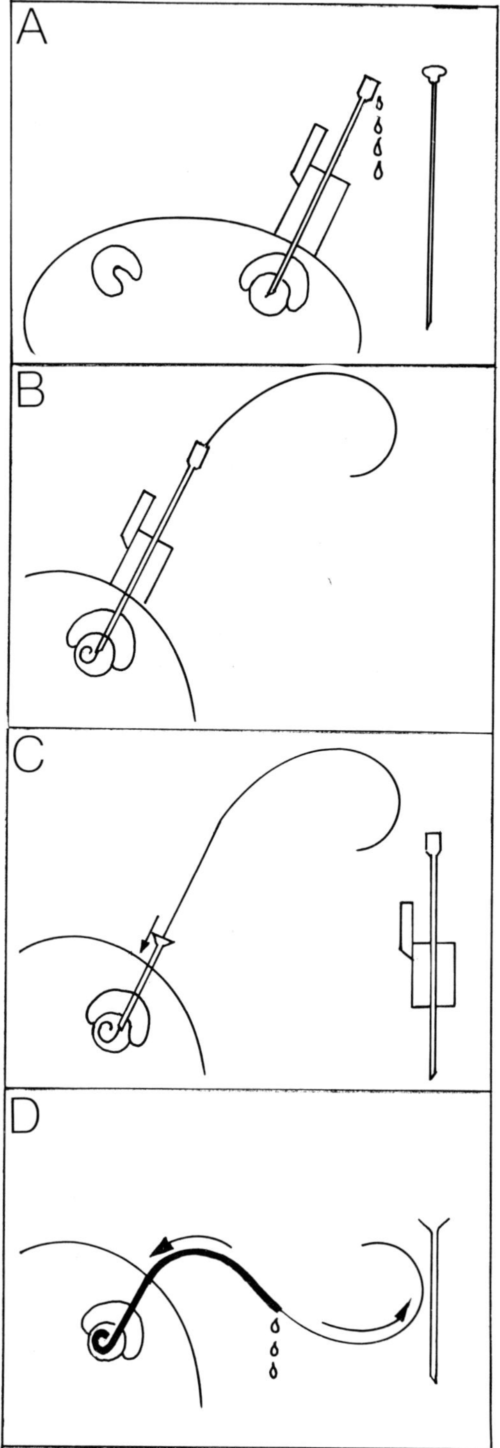

Fig. 9.3. *The procedure of ultrasonically guided nephrostomy*
A. Lumbar needle inserted through puncture transducer into dilated renal pelvis. B. Guide wire passed through needle into pelvis. C. Needle-transducer assembly withdrawn and dilating catheter passed over guide wire into pelvis. D. Soft polyethylene nephrostomy catheter placed into renal pelvis, wire being removed.



Nephrostomy

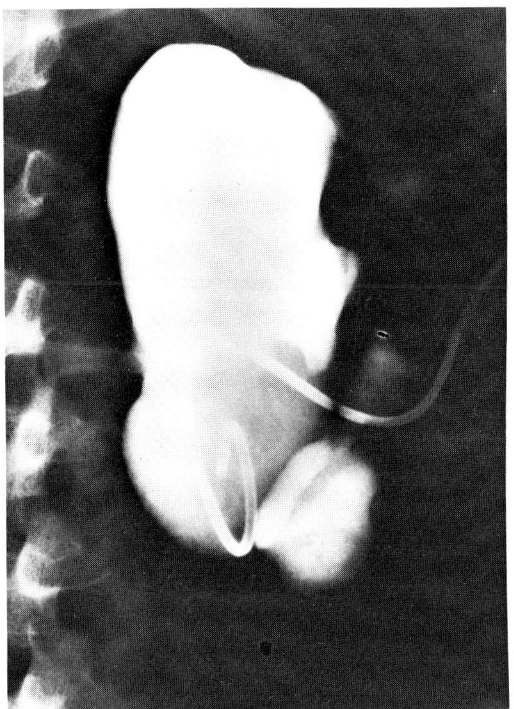

Fig. 9.4. *Antegrade pyelogram*
A coiled catheter in dilated renal pelvis.

renal pelvis 1–48 hours later, preventing long-term drainage or completion of radiographic contrast evaluation. Eight attempts were failures.

The age of the patients ranged from 3 months to 82 years, and the size of the punctured pelves ranged from less than 2 cm to around 10 cm. It is not surprising that the failures as well as the early dislocations occurred mainly in cases of pelves no larger than 2–3 cm.

The number of failures was reduced with the introduction of the short, stiff dilating catheter not used in the early cases. In order to prevent the nephrostomy catheter from slipping out of the pelvis with respiratory motion or patient movement, the catheter should be advanced as far as possible into the renal pelvis.

Bleeding from the renal parenchyma caused no major problems, probably because of the small dimension of the puncturing needle. Furthermore, the somewhat thicker drainage tube will block the puncture canal, thereby also preventing urinary leakage.

Macroscopic hematuria is quite common in the first hours after the catheter placement. Occasionally a 1–3 cm hematoma has been revealed at the kidney convexity at subsequent elective surgery. There was only one significant complication in this series: a perirenal abscess requiring surgical intervention developed after drainage of an infected hydronephrosis.

## Indications

Ultrasonically guided nephrostomy represents a simple and gentle means of placing a nephrostomy tube for therapeutic as well as for diagnostic purposes. The procedure requires only local anesthesia and involves only minimal trauma, which will not interfere with possible later corrective surgery. Given the atraumatic nature, there are several indications for percutaneous nephrostomy:

1. Uremia with ureteral obstruction where retrograde passage of a catheter has failed to bypass the obstruction. The uremia will resolve or at least improve and time be gained for radiographic evaluation and for strategy planning. However, with advanced pelvic malignancy there should be a prospect of response to chemotherapy or radiotherapy before one interferes and resolves the uremia.

2. Infected hydronephrosis causing fever and sepsis. In spite of the risk of spreading the infection, percutaneous drainage is most rewarding by alleviating the toxic symptoms and providing a specimen for culture.

3. To enable antegrade pyelography in obstructive hydronephrosis when intravenous and retrograde pyelography have been unsatisfactory or impossible.

4. In obstructive hydronephrosis temporary percutaneous drainage will show the maximum obtainable function of that kidney, and thus indicate whether corrective surgery or nephrectomy is appropriate.

Other possible indications for percutaneous nephrostomy are:

5. Pelvis irrigation with alkaline fluid to dissolve uric acid calculi.

6. Local chemotherapy of pelvic or ureteral tumors, especially in case of a solitary kidney.

# References


Almgård, L. E. and Fernström I.: Percutaneous nephropyelostomy. *Acta Radiol. (Diagn.) (Stockh.)* 15:288, 1974.

Barbaric, Z. L., Davis, R. S., Frank, I. N., Linke, C. A., Lipchik, E. O. and Crockett, A. T. K.: Percutaneous nephropyelostomy in the management of acute pyohydronephrosis. *Radiol.* 118:567, 1976.

Fowler, J. E., Jr., Meares, E. M., Jr. and Goldin, A. R.: Percutaneous nephrostomy: techniques, indications, and results. *Urol.* 6:428, 1975.

Goodwin, W. E., Casey, W. C. and Woolf, W.: Percutaneous trocar (needle) nephrostomy in hydronephrosis. *J. Am. Med. Assoe.* 157:891, 1955.

Link, D., Leff, R. G., Hildel, J. and Drago, J. R.: The use of percutaneous nephrostomy in 42 patients. *J. Urol.* 122:9, 1979.

Pedersen, J. F.: Percutaneous nephrostomy guided by ultrasound. *J. Urol.* 112:157, 1974.

Pedersen, J. F., Cowan, D. F., Kristensen, J. K., Holm, H. H., Hancke, S. and Jensen, F.: Ultrasonically-guided percutaneous nephrostomy. *Radiol.* 119:429, 1976.

Perinetti, E., Catalona, W. C., Manley, C. B., Geise, G. and Fair, W. R.: Percutaneous nephrostomy: indications, complications and clinical usefulness. *J. Urol.* 120:156, 1978.

Stables, D. P., Ginsberg, N. J. and Johnson, M. L.: Percutaneous nephrostomy: a series and review of the literature. *Am. J. Roentgenol.* 130:75, 1978.

Weinstein, B. J. and Skolnick, M. L.: Ultrasonically guided antegrade pyelography. *J. Urol.* 120:323, 1978.

# CHAPTER X

# Ultrasonically guided renal biopsy

Jørgen Kvist Kristensen

In acute renal insufficiency and in gradually developing impaired renal function, renal biopsy is mandatory in order to obtain a diagnosis upon which a possible specific treatment can be based and in order to set the prognosis for the renal disorder and possibly for the patient. In the end stage of chronic renal insuffiency with contracted kidneys and in polycystic kidney disease biopsy should not be performed since it is without consequences for the treatment and the prognosis is well known. Frequently hypertension is present in this type of renal disorder and it should be kept in mind that severe hypertension is a contraindication for renal biopsy.

Ultrasound has the special advantage in renal biopsy guidance that it visualizes the kidneys, irrespective of their functional capacity. This also means that a morphologic diagnosis of contracted and polycystic kidneys can be made noninvasively.

Before biopsy the patient should be checked for coagulation disorders. He should be fasting overnight and cross-matched blood be available because the procedure carries a certain risk of renal damage with major bleeding requiring surgical intervention.

For the biopsy the patient is placed in the prone position with a sandbag or an inflatable pillow under the abdomen. This is done to avoid anterior displacement of the kidney with the biopsy needle. In addition this procedure improves the ultrasonic visualization of the kidneys. Initially both kidneys are scanned to obtain a morphological diagnosis.

Usually the right kidney is chosen for biopsy because it is the more caudal of the two, which makes access distal to the 12th rib easier. When the kidney for biopsy has been decided upon, it is scanned with the purpose of establishing the optimum site and direction for the introduction of the biopsy needle into the lower part of the kidney. When choosing the direction it is best to introduce the needle perpendicularly to the long axis of the kidney. This gives the best chance of entering the kidney instead of sliding off tangentially because of an oblique angle of introduction.

The lower part is chosen because of the easier access distal to the ribs and to avoid needling of large structures centrally in the renal sinus.

The biopsy may be performed without the use of the biopsy transducer. The needle is directed approximately 2 cm cranial to the lower pole and a point just lateral to the calyceal echoes is chosen. With this direction the distance from the skin to the anterior border of the kidney is read and marked on the biopsy needle. Also the inclination of the scanning plane in relation to the horizontal plane is read. On these premises a thin "pilot" needle is introduced, and when it has entered the kidney, it will be seen to move in synchrony with the respiration of the patient. When the correct direction has been ascertained in this way, the biopsy needle is introduced along the "pilot" needle and the biopsy is performed according to the technique required for the needle type chosen. This depends on individual preferences.

When the biopsy is to be performed with the use of the biopsy transducer, the scanning plane which contains the optimum site and direction for the biopsy is found by scanning with the ordinary transducer. With the static or dynamic biopsy transducer a repeat scan is obtained in this plane and guided by the scan on the screen and the visualized sound beam, the biopsy is performed. Prior to the biopsy a small incision should be made in the skin for easier introduction of the needle.

It takes only a couple of biopsies to get accustomed to performing them via the biopsy transducer and especially with small kidneys the placement of the needle in the kidney is more accurate with this technique. From a theoretical point of view longitudinal position of the scanner is preferable because it may allow the needle in the biopsy transducer to follow possible respiratory kidney displacement.

The biopsy core obtained is examined immediately under a stereo microscope to assure that a sufficient number of glomeruli is present in the specimen, otherwise the procedure is repeated right away.

For final evaluation the biopsy specimen is examined by light microscopy, possibly also with immunofluorescent techniques and electron microscopy, and this requires a good deal of tissue.

After the biopsy the patient is checked regularly and kept in bed until the next day. Microscopic hematuria is a frequent finding after renal biopsy, but usually without clinical significance. Major bleeding into the urinary system or extrarenally may occur and may require surgery, possibly nephrectomy. Although the use of a biopsy transducer makes the system rather rigid, bleeding complications seem not to have increased with the advent of ultrasound guidance, whereas the inadvertent needling of other organs has probably been reduced.

The success rate in obtaining renal tissue using ultrasound guidance is reported to be 95%. This is in accordance with a personal series of 25 patients from whom renal tissue was obtained in 24 cases. In eight of these the serum creatinine was too high to allow fluoroscopic visualization of the kidney after the administration of a radiopaque medium.

The technique is advocated for both the pediatric and adult patient groups.

# References


Bahlmann, J. and Otto, P.: Perkutane Nierenbiopsie mit Ultrashall-Lokalisation. *Dtsch. med. Wschr.* 97:840, 1972.

Bolton, W. K., Tully, R. J., Lewis, E. J. and Ranniger, K.: Localization of the kidney for percutaneous biopsy. *Ann. Int. Med.* 81:159, 1974.

Kristensen, J. K., Bartels, E. and Jørgensen, H. E.: Percutaneous renal biopsy under the guidance of ultrasound. *Scand. J. Urol. Nephrol.* 8:223, 1974.

Mailloux, L. U., Mossey, R. T., McVicar, M. M., Bluestone, P. A. and Goldberg, H. M.: Ultrasonic guidance for renal biopsy. *Arch. Int. Med.* 138:438, 1978.

Mets, T., Lameire, N., Matthys, E. and Afschrift, M.: Sonically guided renal biopsy. *J. Clin. Ultrasound* 7:190, 1979.

Pollack, H. M., Goldberg, B. B. and Kellerman, E.: Ultrasonically guided renal biopsy. *Arch. Int. Med.* 138:355, 1978.

Zeis, P. M., Spigos, D., Samayoa, C., Capek, V. and Aschinberg, L. C.: Ultrasound localization for percutaneous renal biopsy in children. *J. Pediat.* 89:263, 1976.




Renal biopsy

# CHAPTER XI

# Ultrasonic real-time guidance for percutaneous puncture in urology

Masahito Saitoh, Hiroki Watanabe and Hiroshi Ohe

Recent ultrasonic technology has provided rapid advancement in real-time scanners of compact size producing excellent real-time images. A special puncture attachment fastened to the ultrasonic sector scanner was originally developed at our clinic in 1978.

For our first trial an electronic linear scanner was used. However, when a needle was guided obliquely from one end of this type of scanner, a large skin area was required for contact, and there was a considerable distance from the skin surface to the target. Puncture was occasionally made impossible by the ribs or the iliac bone. For those reasons, the sector scanner was thought to be more suitable because of its more compact size and the smaller contact area required. With this type of scanner, the interference from the ribs or the iliac bone was minimized and the distance between the skin and the target was shortened.

A special attachment for needle guidance connected to the sector scanner was then developed. With this equipment the needle is clearly visualized while advanced towards the target.

Echoes from the needle are sufficient for recognition even in solid masses.

Needling under ultrasonic real-time guidance of the kidney, the bladder and the prostate has been carried out at our clinic. A high level of practicability has been demonstrated in all puncture techniques.

## EQUIPMENT

A mechanical sector scanner (ALOKA ASU-25-7C) equipped with a single transducer emitting 3.5 MHz ultrasound is used for ultrasonic real-time imaging (Fig. 11.1). Pendulumlike movements of the transducer produce a real-time sector image. The display speed can be varied from 10 to 30 frames per second. The display angle is also variable, from 30 to 90 degrees. For needling gui-

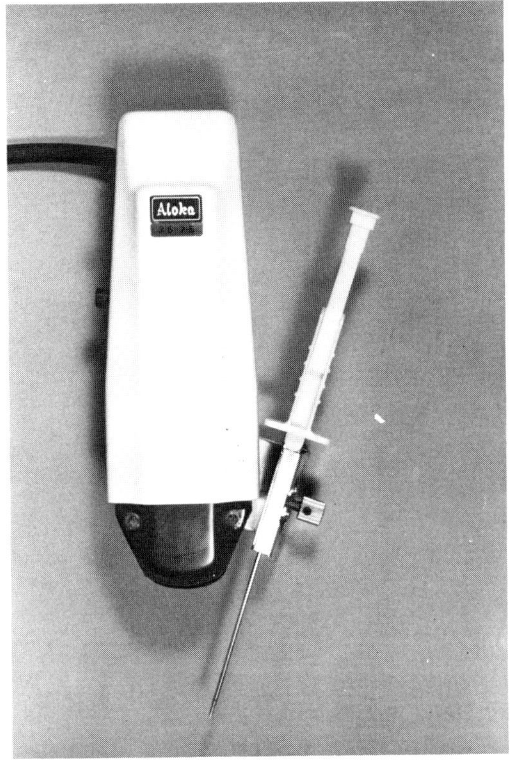

Fig. 11.1. *The dynamic puncture equipment*
Anterior view of the mechanical sector scanner equipped with puncture attachment. The attachment guides a Tru-cut biopsy needle at an oblique angle.

dance, a special attachment made of stainless steel has been developed (Fig. 11.2) which can be easily connected to the scanner. The needle is guided by the attachment into the scanning plane and crosses the longitudinal axis of the scanner at an angle of 20 degrees 8 cm from the skin (Fig. 11.3). By selecting the supplementary metal fitting with a suitable guidance canal, various kinds of needles can be used. When the needle reaches the target, the needle can be released from the attachment

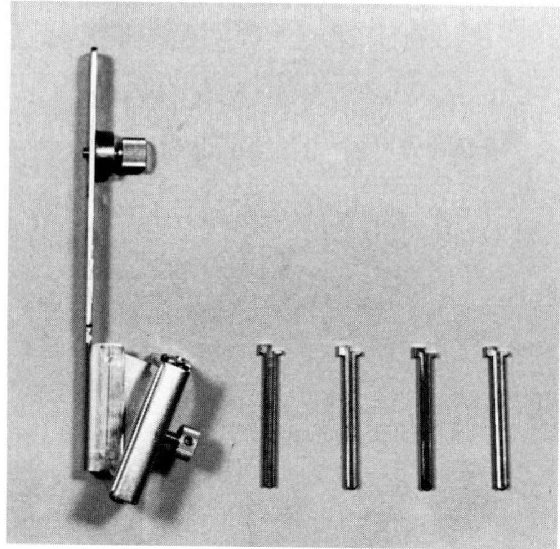

Fig. 11.2. *The puncture attachment*
The attachment and several kinds of supplementary metal fittings with guidance canals.

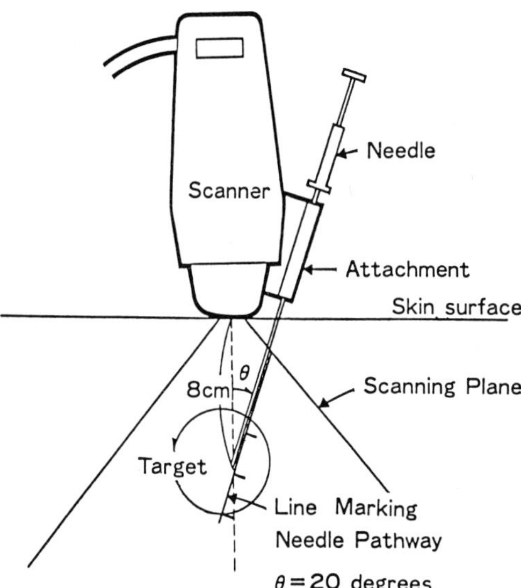


Fig. 11.3. *The needle pathway*
The puncture needle crosses the longitudinal axis of the scanner at an angle of 20 degrees, 8 cm from the skin. The needle pathway is marked on the oscilloscope.

(Fig. 11.4). This causes no interference with the subsequent manipulations (i.e. biopsy, aspiration or tubing).

The needle pathway is marked as an oblique line on the oscilloscope. The needle can be observed advancing along this line.

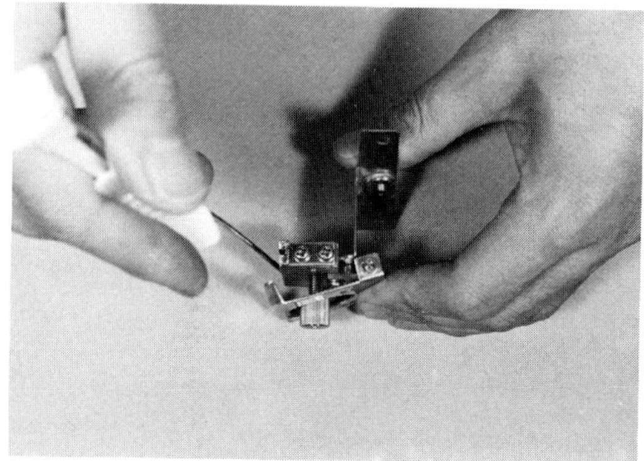

Fig. 11.4. *Needle release*
By opening the metal cover of the attachment, the needle can be released easily.

## PREPARATION AND PROCEDURE

Routine ultrasonic evaluation to assess the target must be made prior to puncture.

Antibiotics and hemostatics may be administered, usually from one day before to several days after puncture.

The attachment is sterilized by autoclave and the scanner is placed overnight in a box filled with formaline gas. If punctures must be performed repeatedly on the same day, the skin contact area of the scanner can be sterilized by 0.5% chlorhexidine-gluconate-alcohol after each use.

The patient is prone for puncture of the kidney and a small pillow may be placed under the abdomen to press the kidney posteriorly. The patient is supine for puncture of the bladder. For puncture of the prostate, the patient is in the lithotomy position. The skin is sterilized and sterile jelly is used as acoustic coupling medium. The puncture attachment is mounted on the scanner. The supplementary metal fitting appropriate to the needle size is placed into the basic canal of the attachment. By changing the position or the angle of the scanner, the puncture site is selected so that the line marking the needle pathway on the oscilloscope traverses the target.

Local anesthetic is injected at this site. The puncture is then performed. The patient is asked to hold his breath until the needle has reached the target. When the needle is in the target the scanner is released from the needle and the subsequent manipulations can be performed unrestricted.



Real-time guidance in urology

# CLINICAL APPLICATIONS

## Kidney

The ultrasonically guided puncture technique is useful for renal biopsy, renal cyst puncture, antegrade pyelography and percutaneous nephrostomy.

### Selective renal biopsy

It is of importance that clear real-time ultrasonograms of the kidney are produced prior to biopsy. Biopsy is made usually with a longitudinal scan. The normal kidney is ovoid. The renal parenchyma is acoustically homogenous and produces few reflections at normal sensitivity levels. Many reflections originate from the structures of the calyces, pelvis and large vessels which are located in the central portion of the kidney.

The central echoes should be avoided when the puncture is made, so that hematuria or gross bleeding into the retroperitoneal space does not occur.

A Tru-cut needle is used. The most common site for routine biopsy is illustrated in Fig. 11.5. In diseases involving the renal medulla (i.e. pyelonephritis, lower nephron nephrosis), the line mark must be positioned very close to the lower margin of the central echoes to obtain a specimen from the renal medulla as well.

The scanner is fixed on the skin so that the line mark on the oscilloscope points to the correct site for biopsy. When the biopsy needle approaches the kidney, the patient should be asked to hold his breath. The interior cutting needle is then advanced. The tip of the needle produces particularly strong reflections and the depth of the insertion can be defined clearly. After the insertion of the interior needle, the scanner is released from the needle and the biopsy performed.

During a 10-month period, 26 selective renal biopsies were performed in 19 adult patients. Tables 11.1 and 11.2 summarize our results.

Renal tissue was obtained from all the patients (100%); 25 specimens were adequate for diagnosis (96%). Renal tissue was not obtained in four puncture attempts (13%) in three patients. The cause of these failures was thought to be that the kidney slipped away because the needle had been directed at too low a section of it. In the following

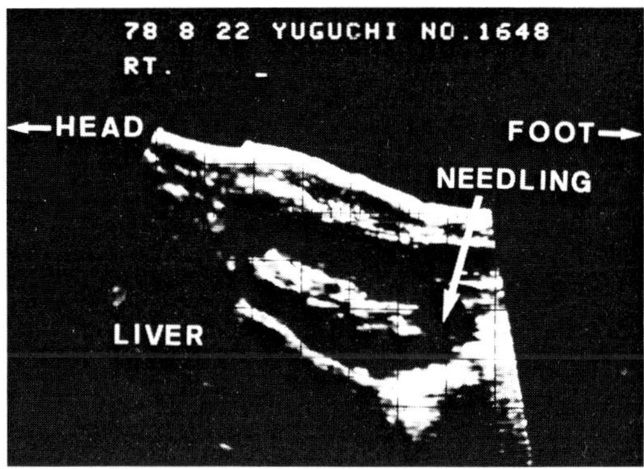


Fig. 11.5. *The most common site for routine renal biopsy* The line mark must be positioned closer to the lower margin of the central echoes when the renal medulla is to be obtained.

Table 11.1. *Results of selective renal biopsy*

| | |
|---|---|
| Patients | 19 |
| Procedures | 26 |
| The kidney chosen for biopsy | |
|     Left | 14( 74%) |
|     Right | 5( 26%) |
| Tissue obtained | 26(100%) |
| Adequate for diagnosis | 25( 96%) |
| Major complication | 0 |

Table 11.2. *Histological diagnosis in 19 patients who had selective renal biopsy performed*

| | |
|---|---|
| Glomerulonephritis | 12 |
| Lupus nephritis | 1 |
| Amyloidosis | 1 |
| Diabetic nephrosis | 1 |
| Chronic pyelonephritis | 2 |
| Normal kidney | 1 |
| Inadequate tissue for diagnosis | 1 |

attempts, however, sufficient specimens were obtained.

As the whole puncture procedure can be monitored in real-time cross-sectional images (Figs. 11.6 and 11.7), there is no danger of injury to the other organs close to the kidney. Both kidneys are therefore available for biopsy. If there were no

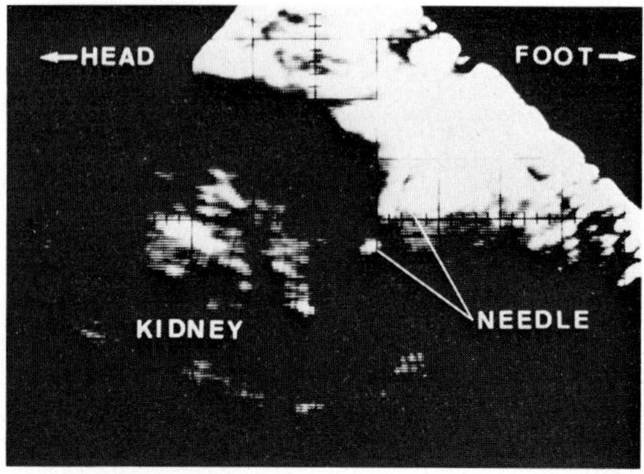


Fig. 11.6. *Percutaneous renal biopsy*
The entire image of a Tru-cut biopsy needle introduced into the parenchyma in the lower pole can be seen clearly. Renal medulla with cortex was obtained in this procedure.

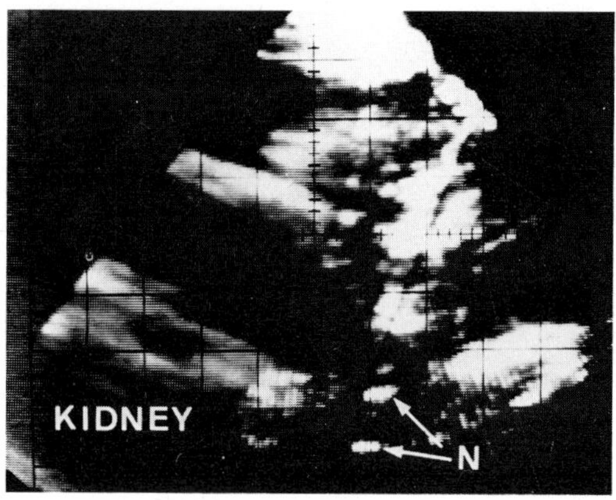


Fig. 11.7. *Percutaneous renal biopsy*
Renal cortex mainly was obtained in this procedure.

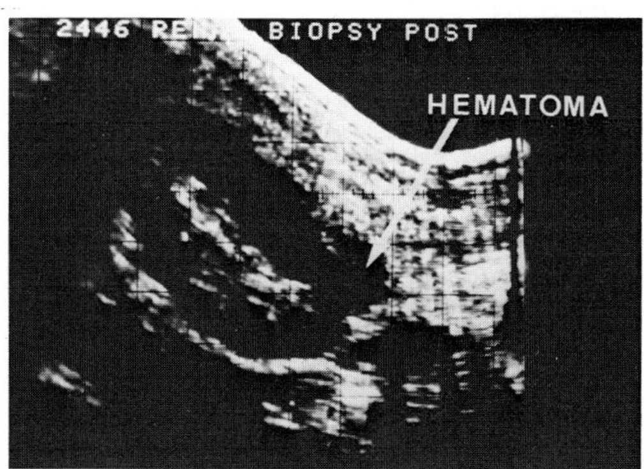


Fig. 11.8. *Retroperitoneal hematoma*
A small retroperitoneal hematoma has been detected by a follow up ultrasonic examination at the puncture site of the kidney.

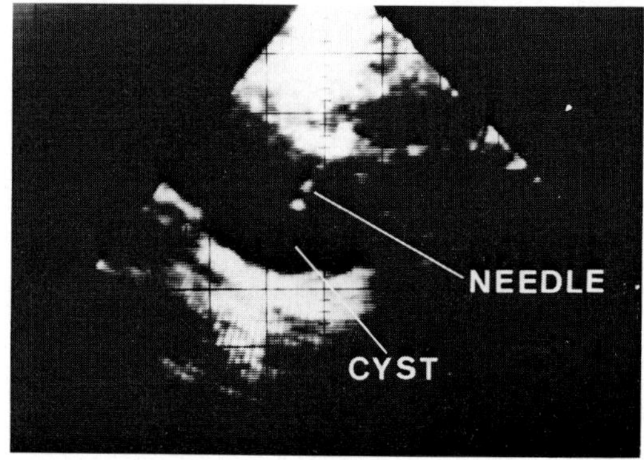


Fig. 11.9. *Renal cyst puncture*
A 21-gauge puncture needle introduced into a cyst in the lower pole can be clearly seen.

special circumstances, the left kidney was chosen in our series because respiratory movements are less pronounced on the left than on the right and the surgeon usually stands on the left side of the patient.

No serious complications occurred. Only one patient complained of slight fever on the day the biopsy was made and of kidney pain for several days afterwards. A very small retroperitoneal hematoma was found by a follow-up ultrasonic examination. (Fig. 11.8) No incidental hematuria, even microscopic, was encountered.

**Renal cyst puncture**
Renal cyst puncture can be carried out easily (Fig. 11.9). A 21-gauge needle is used. The fluid is aspirated and examined cytologically or by culture. Six renal cysts have been punctured. Neither malignant cells nor infection were noticed in any case. No complications occurred.

**Antegrade pyelography**
This technique is useful in cases of hydronephrosis when retrograde pyelography has failed. The dilated renal pelvis is visualized as an echo-free region in the central renal echoes (Fig. 11.10). Sufficient contrast medium is injected through a 21-gauge needle guided into the pelvis (Fig. 11.11). Four cases have been successfully investigated. The causes of hydronephrosis in these cases were tumor invasion of the ureter in three cases and tuberculosis in one. No complications occurred.



Real-time guidance in urology

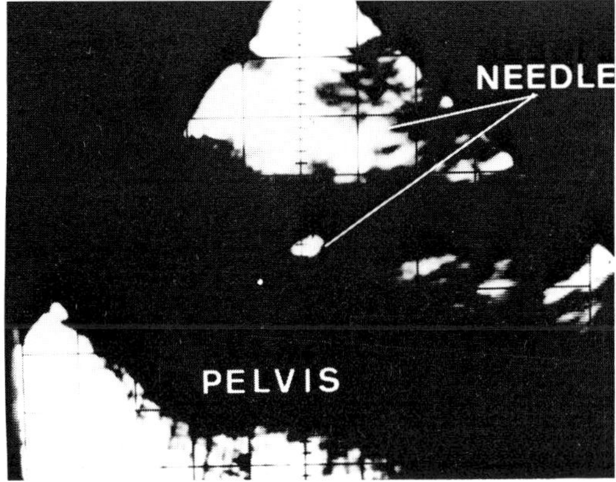

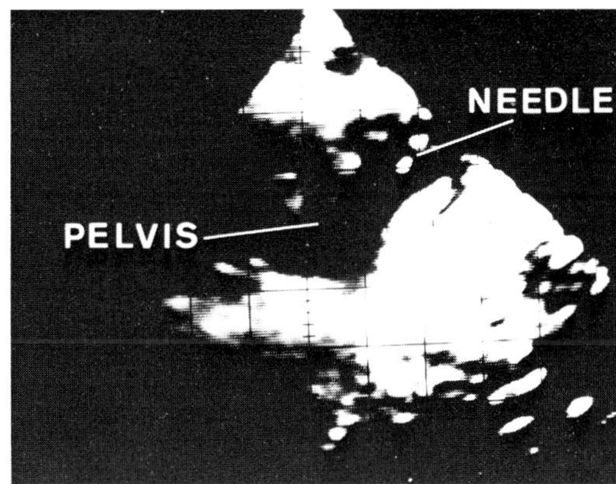



Fig. 11.10. *Antegrade pyelography*
The puncture needle is introduced from the lower pole into the dilated pelvis.

Fig. 11.12. *Percutaneous nephrostomy*
The puncture needle approaches the dilated pelvis. A polyethylene tube was placed in the pelvis through the needle.

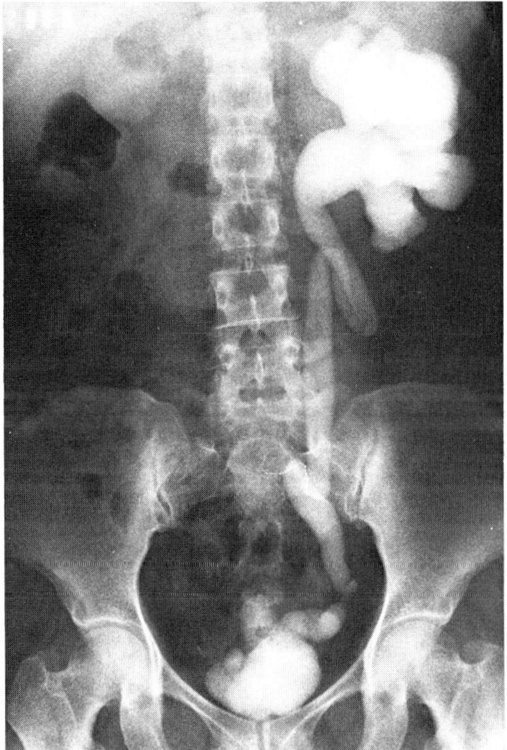

Fig. 11.11. *Antegrade pyelography obtained under real-time guidance.*

## Percutaneous nephrostomy

A polyethylene tube of 1.5 mm diameter is placed in the dilated pelvis through a disposable biopsy needle which has been guided by ultrasound (Fig. 11.12). Urine is drained through the tube con-

tinuously. The Seldinger technique as described by Pedersen has also been used. Three cases have been treated. The causes of the diseases in these three cases were diabetes insipidus, hydronephrosis due to the invasion of a malignant tumor and congenital nephrosis, respectively. Transient macroscopic hematuria was noticed in one case in this series.

## Bladder

### Percutaneous cystostomy

This was successfully performed in a case with urinary retention due to urethral stricture. The technique is the same as for nephrostomy.

### Removal of balloon catheter

Urologists sometimes encounter the difficulty that a balloon catheter placed in the bladder cannot be taken out because of blockage to the water tube. The trouble can be resolved easily by suprapubic puncture of the balloon under ultrasonic real-time guidance.

### Suprapubic bladder aspiration

Goldberg has described ultrasonically guided suprapubic bladder aspiration in newborn babies and young children to obtain an uncontaminated urine sample.

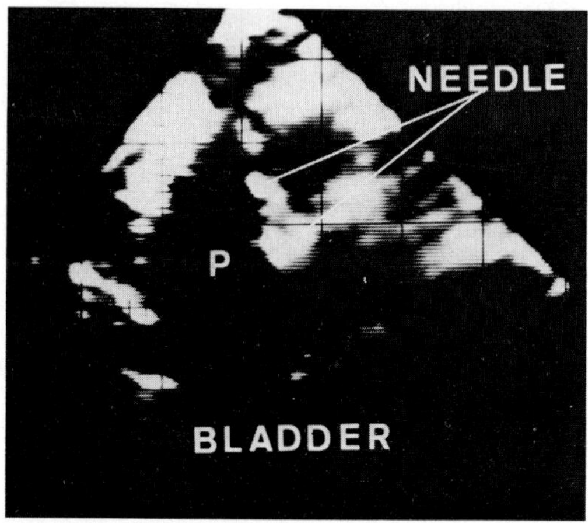


Fig. 11.13. *Perineal prostatic biopsy*
The prostate with a biopsy needle and the bladder are displayed transperineally.

## Prostate

Prostatic biopsy is performed very frequently in urology. Ultrasonic real-time guidance is also applied to perineal prostatic biopsy. By sector scanning it is possible from the perineum to examine the position and the size of the prostate. The puncture technique is the same as mentioned above. A disposable Tru-cut needle is used. Five cases have been investigated (Fig. 11.13). Prostatic cancer in two cases and benign prostatic hypertrophy in three cases were revealed histologically.

However, the prostate is easily palpable from the rectum and ordinary prostatic biopsy can be performed by the guidance of palpation almost without risk or failure. Ultrasonic guidance for biopsy may, accordingly, be less valuable for the prostate than for the kidney.

Ultrasonic real-time guidance is useful, not only in urology but also for general purposes and can be applied to various organs or lesions if they can be visualized by ultrasound. The technique described here provides ideal guidance for needling.


## References

Goldberg, B. B. and Pollack, H. M.: Ultrasonic aspiration transducer. *Radiol* 102:187, 1972.

Goldberg, B. B. and Meyer, H.: Ultrasonically guided suprapubic urinary bladder aspiration. *Pediatrics* 51:70, 1973.

Goldberg, B. B., Pollack, H. M. and Kellerman, E.: Ultrasonic localization for renal biopsy. *Radiol.* 115:167, 1975.

Holm, H. H., Kristensen, J. K., Rasmussen, S. N., Northeved, A. and Barlebo, H.: Ultrasound as a guide in percutaneous puncture technique. *Ultrasonics* 10:83, 1972.

Kristensen, J. K., Bartels, E. and Jørgensen, H. E.: Percutaneous renal biopsy under the guidance of ultrasound. *Scand. J. Urol. Nephrol.* 8:223, 1974.

Mailloux, L. U., Mossey, R. T., McVicar, M. M., Bluestone, P. A. and Goldberg, H. M.: Ultrasonic guidance for renal biopsy. *Arch. Intern. Med.* 138:438, 1978.

Pedersen, J. F.: Percutaneous nephrostomy guided by ultrasound. *J. Urol.* 112:157, 1974.

Pedersen, J. F.: Percutaneous puncture guided by ultrasonic multitransducer scanning. *J. Clin. Ultrasound* 5:175, 1977.

Saitoh, M., Watanabe, H., Ohe, H., Tanaka, S., Itakura, Y. and Date, S.: Ultrasonically guided puncture technique in urology using real-time scanner. *Jap. J. Urol.* 70:46, 1979.

Saitoh, M., Watanabe, H., Ohe, H., Tanaka, S., Itakura, Y. and Date, S.: Ultrasonic real-time guidance for percutaneous puncture. *J. Clin. Ultrasound* 7:269, 1979.

# CHAPTER XII

# Puncture of pancreatic mass lesions

Søren Hancke and Grete Krag Jacobsen

Using ultrasonic scanning, mass lesions can be outlined and solid tumors (Fig. 12.2) can be differentiated from cysts (Fig. 12.3).

Solid tumors of the pancreas are most often caused either by chronic pancreatitis or carcinomas, while cystic lesions in the majority of cases are caused by pancreatic pseudocysts or abscesses.

When a solid mass lesion of the pancreas is demonstrated ultrasonically it is in most cases not possible from the scans to predict whether the mass is benign or malignant. However, a preoperative cytological diagnosis of malignancy may be obtained through a percutaneous fine needle biopsy guided by ultrasonic scanning.

Pancreatic cysts may also be punctured percutaneously and for this purpose too, ultrasound is perfect for needle guidance.

## ASPIRATION BIOPSY FROM SOLID MASS LESIONS

## Procedure

The patient should be fasting and checked for

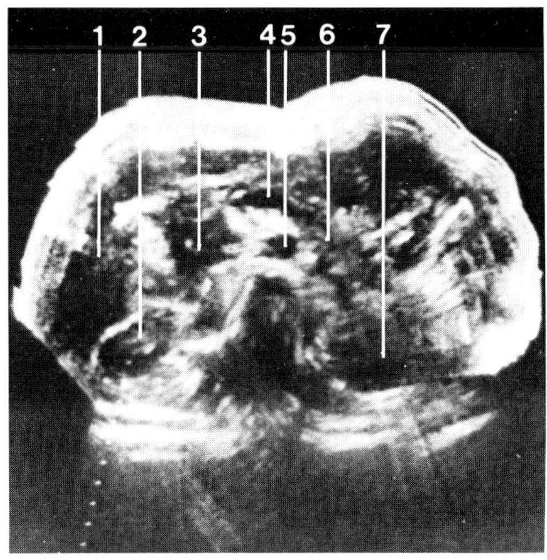

Fig. 12.2. *Carcinoma of the head of the pancreas*
Transverse scan. 1. Liver, 2. Right kidney, 3. Solid mass in the head of the pancreas, 4. Body of pancreas, 5. Aorta, 6. Tail of pancreas, 7. Left kidney.

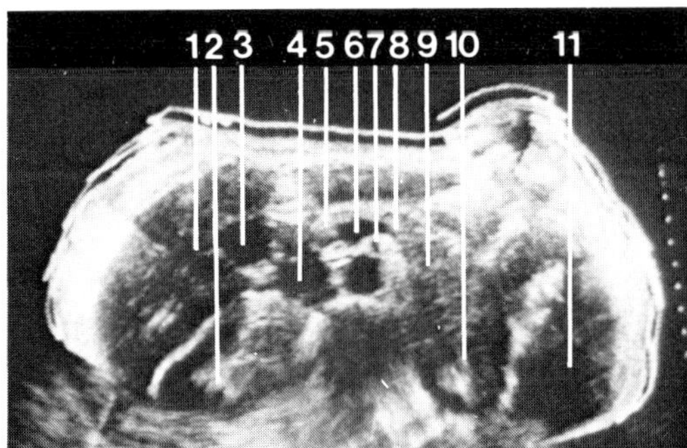

Fig. 12.1. *Normal pancreas*
Transverse scan. 1. Liver, 2. Right kidney, 3. Gall bladder, 4. Inferior vena cava, 5. Head of pancreas, 6. Portal vein, 7. Superior mesenteric artery anterior to the aorta, 8. Body of pancreas, 9. Tail of pancreas, 10. Left kidney, 11. Spleen.

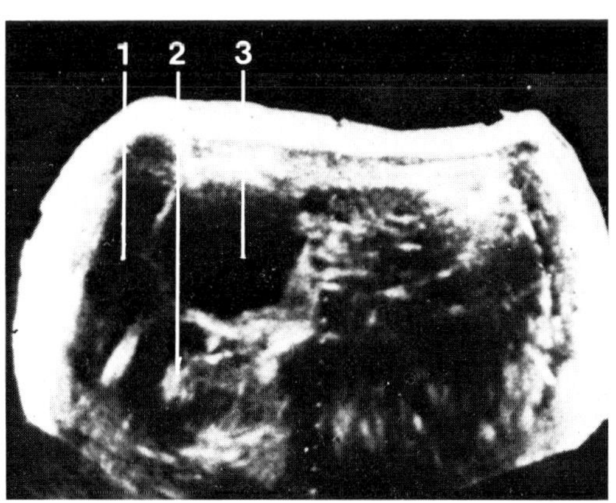

Fig. 12.3. *Pseudocyst in the head of the pancreas*
Transverse scan. 1. Liver, 2. Right kidney, 3. Pancreatic pseudocyst.

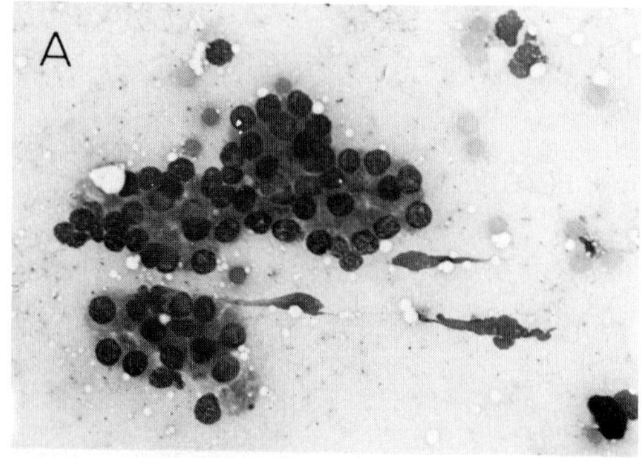

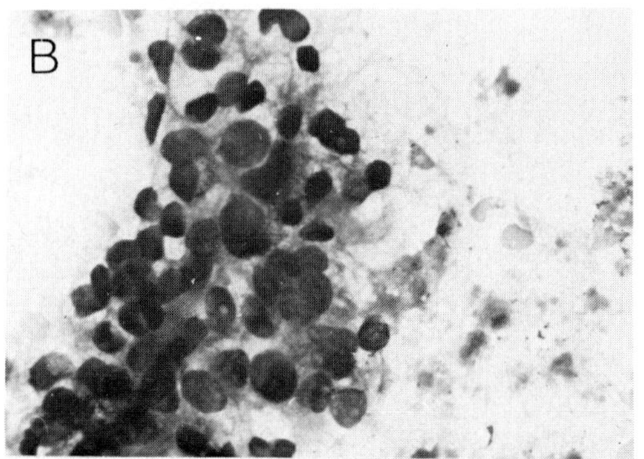

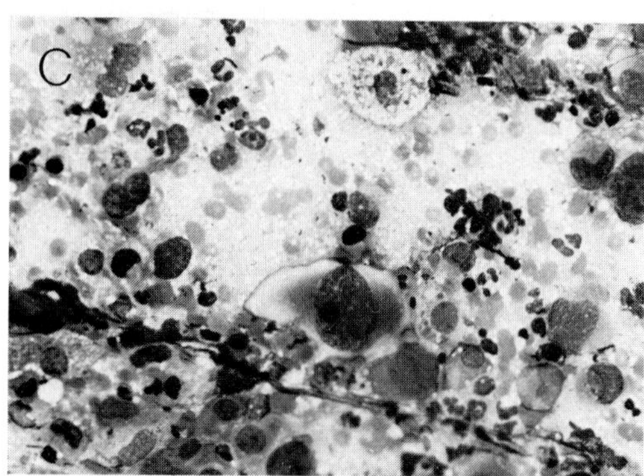

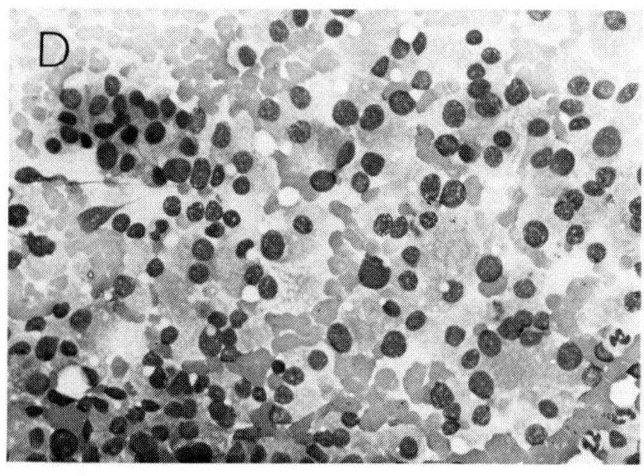

hemorrhagic disorders. From ordinary scans the optimum site and direction for biopsy are established. The gastrointestinal tract can be traversed without harm. In case of a large left lobe of the liver the transhepatic route is acceptable. When the depth and direction have been established, a guide needle is inserted through the biopsy transducer and the abdominal wall exclusively. Through the guide needle the fine needle is introduced into the lesion which is usually felt to be of firm consistency. The aspiration is performed according to the technique described in chapter V. Three to six aspirations with the fine needle through the same guide needle in various directions are usually performed in order to obtain material from various parts of the lesion.

Each aspiration usually contains sufficient material to be expelled onto two to four glass slides with one drop on each slide. One drop is spread into a thin transparent layer between two glass slides givning a total of four to eight slides. The specimens are air dried at room temperature and stained according to May-Grünwald-Giemsa.

It is possible within 30 minutes to examine the aspirates. During that time the patient may stay in the examination room and another biopsy be obtained if the first one does not yield sufficient material for conslusive diagnosis.

## Cytological findings

**Normal pancreas.** An aspirate obtained from the parenchyma of the normal pancreas is usually not

Fig. 12.4. *Pancreatic fine needle biopsy* (May-Grünwald-Giemsa, × 250)
A. *Aspirate from a normal pancreas.*
   A group of normal acinar cells are seen on a slightly blood contaminated but otherwise clean background.
B. *Aspirate from a highly differentiated carcinoma of the pancreas.*
   A thick cluster of cells with moderately pleomorphic nuclei and vacuolated cytoplasma is present on a background with necrotic debris.
C. *Aspirate from a low differentiated carcinoma of the pancreas.*
   Numerous pleomorphic epithelial cells with large nuclei containing conspicuous nucleoli are present, intermingled with necrotic debris and leucocytes.
D. *Aspirate from a tumor of the islets of Langerhans.*
   A cellular aspirate with fairly uniform cells with rounded nuclei surrounded by abundant, slightly stained cytoplasm is demonstrated.

very cellular. It contains acinar and ductal cells and to a lesser degree endothelial and mesenchymal cells (Fig. 12.4 A). Acinar cells appear in small clusters of uniform cells with rosette formations. The ductal cells occur mostly in rather large single-layer sheets with a regular mosaic arrangement of uniform cells. Cells of the islets are seldom seen.

**Pancreatitis.** Material from inflammatory lesions of the pancreas contains some or few acinar and duct cells with normal appearance or with various degrees of inflammatory changes, i.e. slight variations in size and shape of cells and nuclei. Furthermore, conspicious nucleoli may be present. The cell background of the aspirate is fairly characteristic. Numerous inflammatory cells and necrotic debris with both fine and coarse granular appearance are present.

**Carcinomas.** Most cases of pancreatic carcinomas are adenocarcinomas of the exocrine or ductal epithelium. Cells from these tumors fulfill the usual cytological criteria of malignancy and generally, do not present diagnostic problems (Fig. 12.4 B & C). In addition, the cell background in material aspirated from carcinomas will contain necrotic material of coarse granular debris intermingled with tumor cells of varying degrees of degeneration together with some inflammatory cells.

**Tumors of the islets of Langerhans.** This special group of tumors shows a cellular picture which will often be easily recognized (Fig. 12.4 D). The aspirate is usually very cellular and cells are uniform with round nuclei surrounded by abundant, slightly stained cytoplasm.

## Results

In a series of 90 patients in whom ultrasonic scanning showed a solid enlargement of the pancreas, a percutaneous fine needle biopsy was performed. Fifty-three patients had a carcinoma of the pancreas and in 43 of these tumor cells were demonstrated cytologically. Thirty-seven patients did not have a malignant pancreatic disease. No false positive cytological diagnoses of malignancy were made. In two cases cytology was inconclusive. No significant complications were encoun-

tered, neither bleeding, infection nor fistula formation.

## CYST PUNCTURE

## Procedure

To define the optimal site for puncture, transverse and longitudinal scans through the cyst are initially performed. The shortest distance from the skin to the cyst is chosen and the puncture site may be either in the epigastrium or laterally in an intercostal space. The puncture is carried out by means of a 1.2 mm needle. Since the tip of the rather thick needle can be visualized on the scan, the needle may be advanced or withdrawn during aspiration so almost quantitative emptying of the cyst is possible. Part of the gastrointestinal tract may be traversed by the needle, but puncture of the liver should be avoided.

The aspirated fluid of recently developed pancreatic pseudocysts is usually dark, brownish, while the fluid in old cysts or in cysts previously aspirated may be clear yellow. It has usually a high concentration of amylase. An abscess is easily diagnosed if pus is aspirated.

## Cytological findings

For cytological evaluation the cyst fluid is centrifuged and the sediment placed onto glass slides as described previously. After air drying at room temperature the specimens are stained according to May-Grünwald-Giemsa.

Material obtained from cysts contains epithelial cells in varying numbers with varying degrees of degeneration together with protein precipitations and nuclei shadows of disintegrated inflammatory cells. Material from inflammatory cysts or abscesses contains pus with numerous leucocytes and some macrophages.

## Results

A series of 40 patients had an ultrasonically guided pancreatic cyst puncture performed. The size of the cysts ranged from 3 to 20 cm in diameter, 12 of which were smaller than 4 cm. Nine patients had two cysts which were both punctured.

In all cases aspiration was successful. Nine patients were repunctured up to five times. Twenty-one patients had recurrences within a few months, whereas three were without recurrence after 12 months. In three patients radiopaque material was injected. In one of these the contrast medium outlined the ductal system in the tail, but not in the head of the pancreas suggesting a stenosis of the pancreatic duct. In four patients pus was aspirated – a pancreatic abscess was present. The series did not include any malignant cysts.

The punctures were all performed with only slight or no discomfort to the patients. There was only one complication. A 42-year-old female presented with a 200 ml echo-free area at the site of the cyst at follow-up ultrasonic scanning 3 months after cyst aspiration. Operation for recurrence was planned, but at laparotomy the cyst had disappeared. A 200 ml hematoma between the liver and the stomach was found.

A fine needle biopsy should be performed whenever a *solid enlargement of the pancreas* is demonstrated or suspected. Exceptions are patients with acute or relapsing chronic pancreatitis and patients with hemorrhagic diathesis. Patients with jaundice or portal hypertension should not be excluded.

False positive cytological diagnoses have not been encountered in the literature, nor in the present series, giving a diagnostic specificity of 100%. The diagnostic sensitivity is 80–85%. Therefore, absence of malignant cells does not exclude cancer.

One of the reasons for false negative cytological diagnoses may be the fact that pancreatic carcinomas are often surrounded by or contain abundant fibrous tissue from where no malignant cells can be aspirated.

In the literature no false positive diagnoses among 155 punctured benign pancreatic lesions are recorded. One of the reasons for this may be that malignant cells from carcinomas of the pancreas in most cases show obvious signs of malignancy.

Inconclusive cytological diagnoses may be due to disintegrated cells or to the aspiration of very few atypical cells.

In pancreatic diagnosis, percutaneous fine needle biopsy has great advantages. In patients where surgery is indicated, a preoperatively established cancer diagnosis enables the surgeon to perform palliative or radical surgery immediately. A possible risk by intraoperative biopsy and difficulties in the interpretation of frozen sections can be avoided. In some cases a positive biopsy may eliminate the need for surgery. This is the case when the patient is unfit for radical resection and when pain indicates nerve involvement which means inoperability.

Dissemination of tumor cells to the blood or lymph stream or to the needle tract may theoretically occur, but since the prognosis of a pancreatic cancer is extremely poor, the possibility of an early diagnosis or a diagnosis obtained in a gentle manner by far outweighs the theoretical possibility of tumor spread. One must consider that exploratory laparotomy in itself may imply a risk of tumor spread.

When a *cystic mass lesion of the pancreas* is demonstrated ultrasonically, percutaneous aspiration may be performed to provide additional information about the nature of the lesion and also as a therapeutic means. Ultrasonically guided cyst puncture is easy and simple with little risk and discomfort to the patient.

With the aspiration of fluid the ultrasonic diagnosis is verified and through amylase analysis differentiation from other abdominal cysts can be made. If pus is aspirated, an abscess is present and from bacteriological study adequate antibiotic therapy can be established. In cases of threatening rupture of an acutely developed cyst decompression by puncture is advantageous. Repeated puncture may allow time for "maturation" of the cyst membrane, thereby facilitating surgical intervention. A patient who is acutely ill and has a rapidly developing pancreatic pseudocyst can be relieved and time gained to improve his general physical condition. By fluid aspiration from a pancreatic pseudocyst followed by injection of radiopaque material into the cyst, possible communication to the ductal system of the pancreas can be demonstrated, and give valuable information to the surgeon. Rare instances of malignant pancreatic cysts may be disclosed by cytological analysis of the aspirated fluid. Finally, the possibility of definitive therapy through a single or repeated percutaneous puncture exists.

# References


Clouse, M.E., Gregg, J. A., McDonald, D. G. and Legg, M. A.: Percutaneous fine needle aspiration biopsy of pancreatic carcinoma. *Gastrointest. Radiol.* 2:67, 1977.

Goldman, M. L., Naib, Z. M., Galambos, J. T., Rudé, J. C., Oen, K. T., Bradley, E. L., Salam, A. and Gonzales, A. C.: Preoperative diagnosis of pancreatic carcinoma by percutaneous aspiration biopsy. *Digestive Dis.* 22:1076, 1977.

Goldstein, H. M. and Zornoza, J.: Percutaneous transperitoneal aspiration biopsy of pancreatic masses. *Digestive Dis.* 23:840, 1978.

Hancke, S., Holm, H. H. and Koch, F.: Ultrasonically guided percutaneous fine needle biopsy of the pancreas. *Surg. Gynecol. Obstet.* 140:361, 1975.

Hancke, S. and Pedersen, J. F.: Percutaneous puncture of pancreatic cysts guided by ultrasound. *Surg. Gynecol. Obstet.* 142:551, 1976.

McLoughlin, M. J., Ho, C. S., Langer, B., McHattie, J. and Tao, L. C.: Fine needle aspiration biopsy of malignant lesions in and around the pancreas. *Cancer* 41:2413, 1978.

Oscarson, J., Stormby, N. and Sundgren, R.: Selective angiography in fine-needle aspiration cyto-diagnosis of gastric and pancreatic tumors. *Acta Radiol.* 12:737, 1972.

Smith, E. H., Bartrum, R. J., Chang, Y. C., D'Orsi, C. J., Lokich, J., Abbruzzese, A. and Dantone, J.: Percutaneous aspiration biopsy of the pancreas under ultrasonic guidance. *N. Engl. J. Med.* 292:825, 1975.

Tao, L. C., Ho, C. S., Loughlin, M. J. and McHattie, J.: Percutaneous fine needle aspiration biopsy of the pancreas. *Acta Cytol.* 22:215, 1978.

Tylén, U., Arnesjö, B., Lindberg, L. G., Lunderquist, A. and Åkerman, M.: Percutaneous biopsy of carcinoma of the pancreas guided by angiography. *Surg. Gynecol. Obstet.* 142:737, 1976.

# CHAPTER XIII

# Ultrasonically guided liver biopsy and puncture of hepatic mass lesions

Sten Nørby Rasmussen and Ole Boll Henriksen

There are numerous indications for performing percutaneous puncture of the liver. This chapter will deal only with coarse needle biopsy in diffuse liver disease, fine needle biopsy of focal liver lesions and puncture of cystic liver lesions.

## COARSE NEEDLE BIOPSY IN DIFFUSE LIVER DISEASE

Coarse-needle liver biopsy should always be regarded as potentially fatal. The patients must be carefully selected, a real indication must be present, and serum-bilirubin, alkaline phosphatases and serum-alanine-aminotransferases together with an analysis of the coagulation systems, should always be carried out. The patient's blood group should be known and a pint of compatible blood should be available. The aftercare of the patient should be intensive, including monitoring of pulse rate and blood pressure regularly for 24 hours. With such precautions complications will very seldom be seen and fatal cases be fewer than 2%.

In certain situations there is an increased risk in performing liver biopsy:

1) Presence of ascites, in which case the liver may float away from the biopsy needle. Ultrasound can diagnose ascitic fluid, and if biopsy of the liver is still wanted, the fluid may be tapped and its disappearance demonstrated ultrasonically before biopsy.

2) If the liver is small, a traditional "blind" biopsy can miss the liver, and puncture the gall bladder, intestines, kidney or large blood vessels instead.

3) In case the size or shape of the liver is abnormal, the above-mentioned risks are also present.

4) In fat patients, a liver of normal size is often displaced cranially, and percussion is extremely unreliable. When a liver biopsy is attempted in such cases, the liver is often not hit because it is situated cranial to the ordinary site of puncture which is the $8^{th}$ and $9^{th}$ intercostal space in the right midaxillary line.

When such conditions are known or suspected, it is suggested that coarse-needle liver biopsy is performed under the guidance of ultrasonic scanning, simply by the registration of a few longitudinal and transverse scans through the region of the liver, and the optimum site for puncture may then be chosen.

In these situations ultrasonic guidance is mandatory, but actually all liver biopsies ought to be preceded by an ultrasonic "survey" scanning in order to provide as much information as possible about the anatomy of the biopsy region.

## FINE NEEDLE BIOPSY OF FOCAL LIVER LESIONS

In fine needle biopsies of the liver bleeding and coagulation time should be checked and the patient be fasting.

In most cases of focal liver lesions a special puncture transducer is needed to guide the biopsy (see chapter IV).

When verification or exclusion of malignancy in an ultrasonically suspected focal liver lesion is wanted, an ultrasonically guided fine needle aspiration technique is satisfactory (Fig. 13.1). When the aim is to determine the origin of a liver metastasis, an ultrasonically guided coarse needle biopsy – providing a tissue core – is necessary in most cases.

**Liver metastases** are frequent. Ultrasonically they may be of the typical echo-rich type (Fig. 13.2 A) or a central echo-poor area within the echo-rich area may be seen (Fig. 13.2 B). Liver metastases may also be of the echo-poor type (Fig. 13.2 C) and this may be modified by the appearance of a central echo-rich area (Fig. 13.2 D). Finally, liver

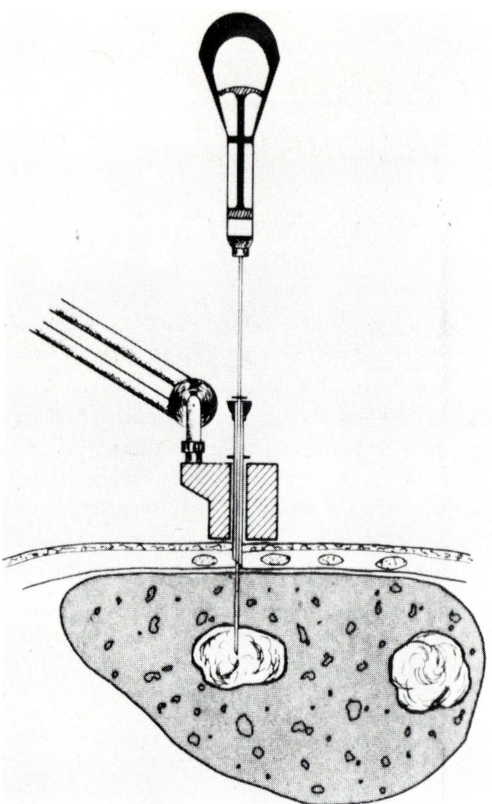

Fig. 13.1. *Ultrasonically guided fine needle biopsy*
Schematic demonstration of the procedure used for ultrasonically guided fine needle aspiration biopsy of focal liver lesions.

metastases sometimes cause echo confirgurations which are a total mixture of all the echo types mentioned (Fig. 13.2 E). Some studies have tried to correlate the site of the primary tumor or its histologic type with the ultrasonic pattern of the metastases. With the exception of leiomyosarcomas which cause typical ultrasonically echo-poor liver lesions sometimes with a sediment (Fig. 13.3 A) and adenocarcinomatous metastases from the large intestine which most frequently are very echo-rich (Fig. 13.3 B), no suggestions concerning histology and site of origin can be obtained from the ultrasonic appearance of liver lesions.

As the diagnostic specificity and sensitivity of an ultrasonic scanning for liver metastases is not sufficiently high, the definite positive diagnosis is still based upon the histologic or cytologic demonstration of tumor tissue or tumor cells.

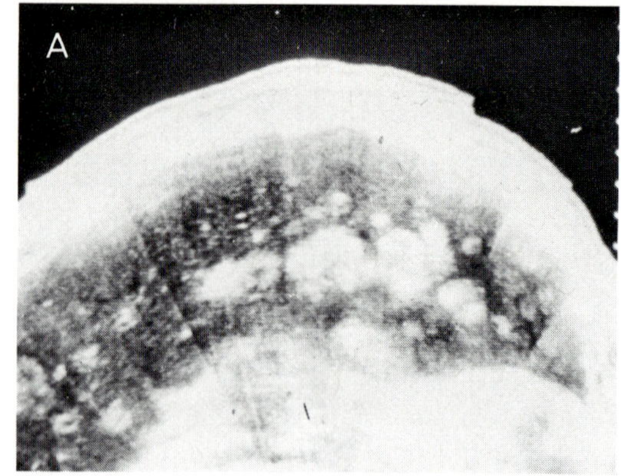

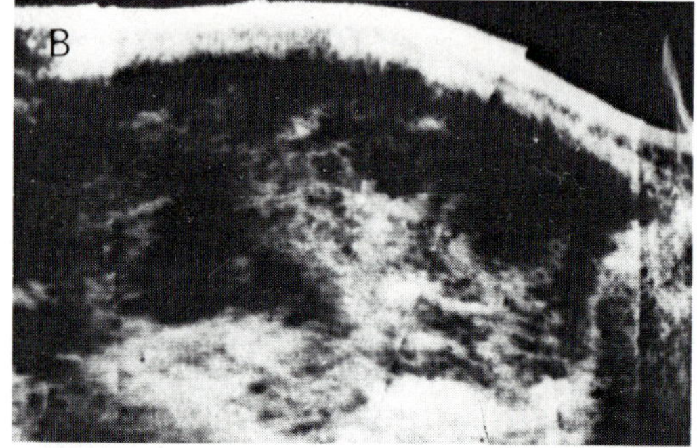

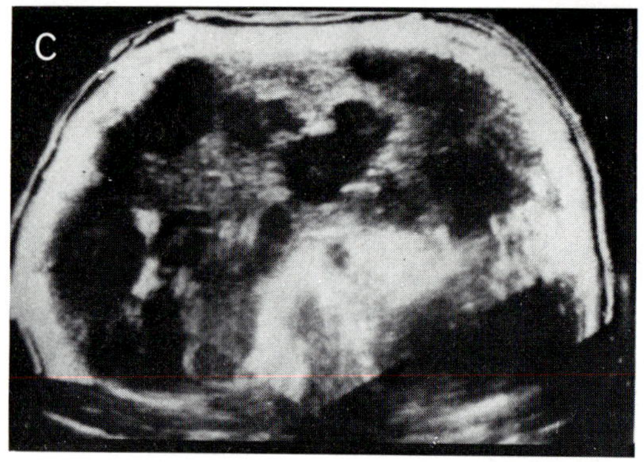

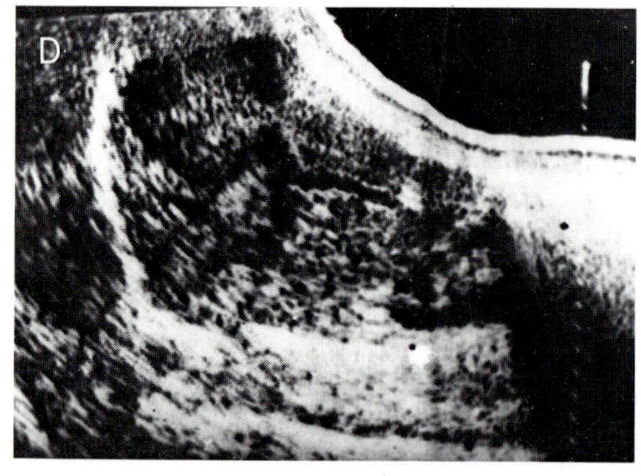

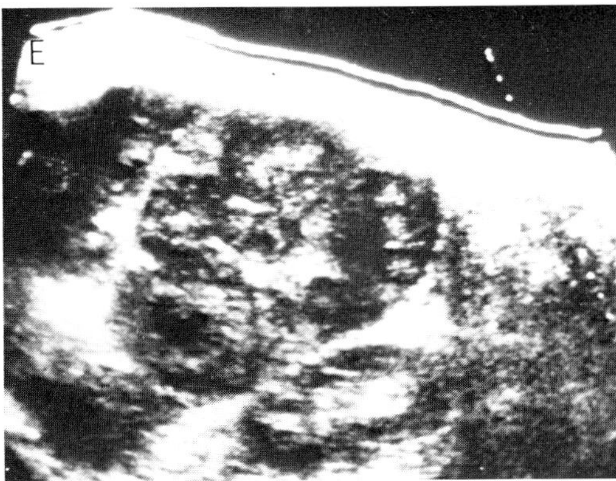

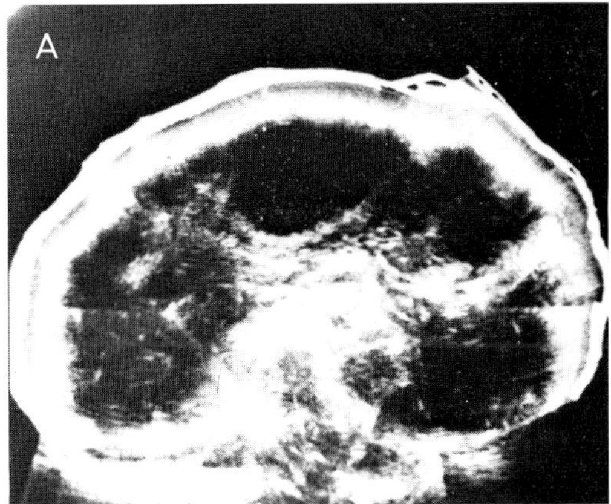

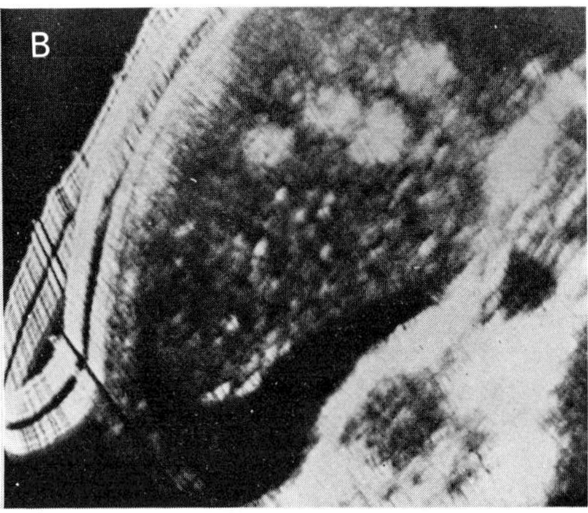

Fig. 13.2. *Liver metastases*
A. Transverse scan, echo-rich metastases. B. Longitudinal scan, echo-rich metastases with echo-poor center. C. Transverse scan, echo-poor metastases. D. Longitudinal scan, echo-poor metastases with echo-rich center. E. Longitudinal scan, metastases representing a mixture of all above-mentioned echo-types.

Fig. 13.3. *Correlation of histology and echo pattern*
A. Transverse scan through liver with several echo-poor lesions representing metastases from a leiomyosarcoma. In the center of the liver is seen a large lesion with a sediment. B. Transverse scan through the right lobe of a liver with four echo-rich metastases from a adenocarcinoma of the colon. Behind the liver, ascites is seen.

In case of ultrasonically suspected metastases, a biopsy with a 0.6 mm needle is performed after the introduction of a guide needle through the abdominal wall only (Fig. 13.1).

In a series of patients with ultrasonically suspected liver metastases, fine needle aspiration biopsy guided by ultrasound was compared to traditional "blind" Menghini biopsy. As could be expected, tumor cells were obtained in a statistically significant higher number of cases with the ultrasonically guided fine needle technique than with the "blind" Menghini technique.

The material from *normal liver aspirates* usually is moderately cellular with scattered groups of liver cells, arranged in rather short bars containing large, polygonal cytoplasm-rich cells with regular nuclei having an evenly distributed chromatin content, sometimes with nucleoli (Fig. 13.4). Within a single group the liver cells may vary a great deal in size . Often small groups of bile epithelium may be seen. These cells are smaller than the liver cells and are of very uniform size.

In cases of *malignancy* necrotic material is often encountered in the aspirate. In addition malignant cells that fulfill the usual criteria of malignancy should be found, either in sheets with irregular shape (Fig. 13.5) or singly, scattered in the material. In cases of metastases from endocrine tumors, the cells are often abundant and rather small with only very slight indication of malignancy, if any. The number of cells and their arrangement in sheets without the regularity usually seen in bile duct epithelium suggest the secondaries to be of endocrine origin.

**Primary liver tumors** such as hepatomas and cholangiogenic carcinomas are often difficult to recognize clinically. Ultrasonically they usually present more echo-rich than the normal liver parenchyma (Fig. 13.6), but these differences between echo-strength may be subtle.

Cytologically they present the usual criteria of malignancy. Most often the cytology does not differ from other malignant carcinomas (Fig. 13.7).

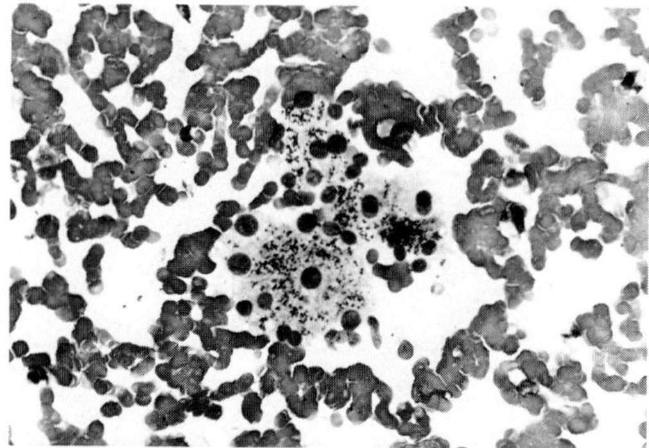

Fig. 13.4. *Aspirate from normal liver parenchyma*
Group of normal liver cells showing some cell and nuclear size variation. The cells have an abundant, often ill-defined cytoplasm which may contain granular material ($\times$ 300).

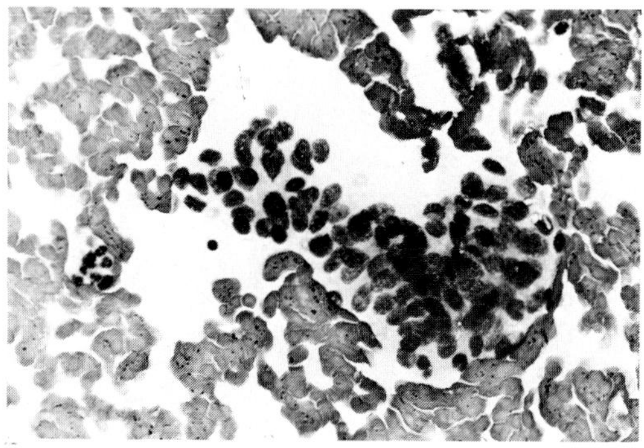

Fig. 13.5. *Aspirate from adenocarcinomatous metastasis*
Sheet of epithelial cells with large hyperchromatic nuclei and rather scanty ill-defined pale cytoplasm, cellular arrangement suggestive of adenocarcinoma (adenocarcinoma of colon) ($\times$ 300).

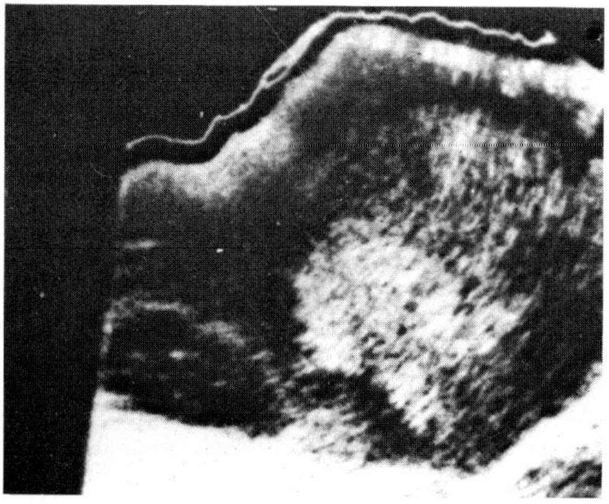

Fig. 13.6. *Primary tumor of the liver*
Longitudinal scan through the right lobe of the liver. A central, echo-rich area is seen representing a hepatoma.

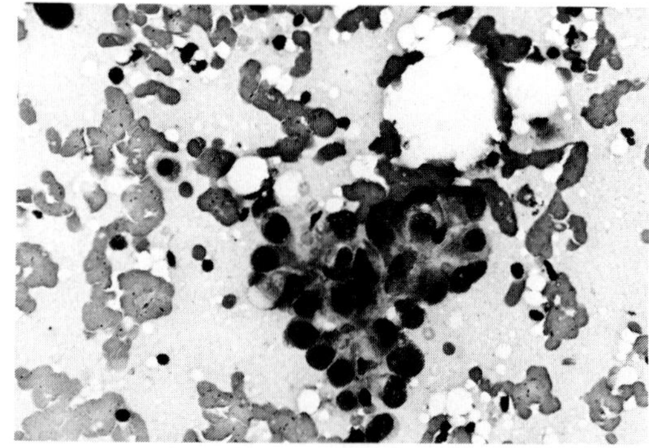

Fig. 13.7. *Aspirate from primary tumor of the liver*
Group of epithelial cells in acinar or adenomatous configuration with varying cell and nuclear size. Nuclei are hyperchromatic and irregular, cytoplasm fairly abundant, suggesting adenocarcinoma (cholangiocarcinoma) ($\times$ 300).

# PUNCTURE OF CYSTIC LIVER LESIONS

While all types of solid liver lesions are potential biopsy targets, this is not the case in all cystic liver lesions.

**Solitary liver cysts** (Fig. 13.8) can be punctured, in most cases to relieve the remaining parenchyma of mechanical pressure. Cytologically the aspirates from liver cysts should contain only very few cells, mostly macrophages.

**Amebic liver abscess** may be suspected with possible exposure of the patient, i.e. geographical history, possibly the demonstration of amebic trophozoites or cysts in stools or rectal curettage, positive serology, and the demonstration on an ultrasound scan of a cystic lesion of the liver (Fig. 13.9). Puncture of such a lesion may be indicated for diagnostic or therapeutic reasons. Typically an amebic liver abscess contains light-brown fluid. Trophozoites are seldom demonstrated in the aspirate. Puncture and emptying of an amebic liver abscess is indicated if the lesion is larger than 5–6 cm in diameter, as this procedure hastens resolution. Provided enteric amebiasis is not present, the patient is treated short-term with metronidazol in a high dose for 24 hours in connection with the puncture in order to avoid hematogenous dissemination. If the abscess has not disappeared at control scan, repuncture may be performed several times.

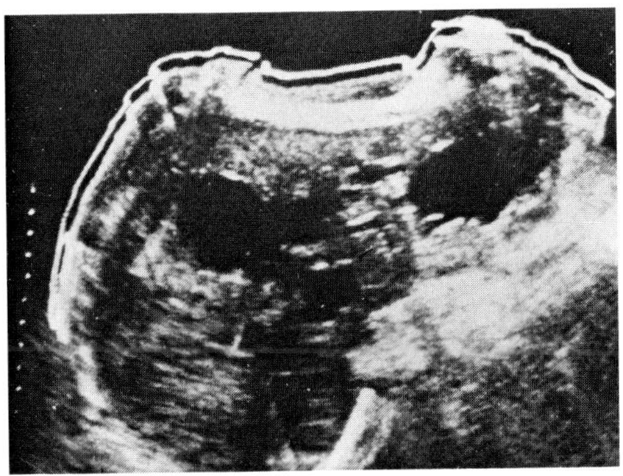

Fig. 13.8. *Liver cysts*
Transverse scan through liver with two echo-poor lesions representing liver cysts.

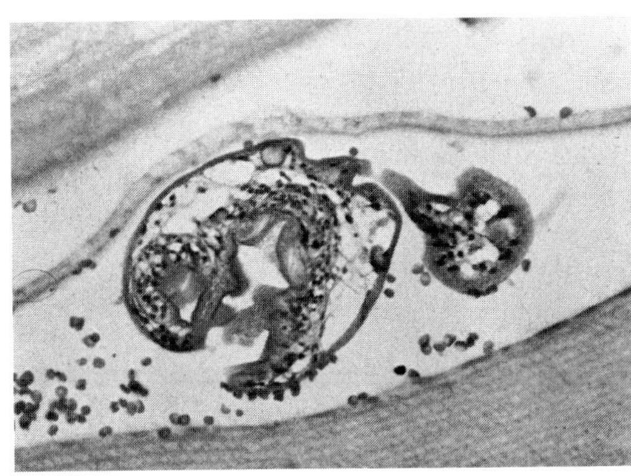

Fig. 13.10. *Scolex of hydatid cyst*
The scolex is seen invaginated in its own cyst membrane so that hooklets and suckers are faced inwards in order to protect them from injury.

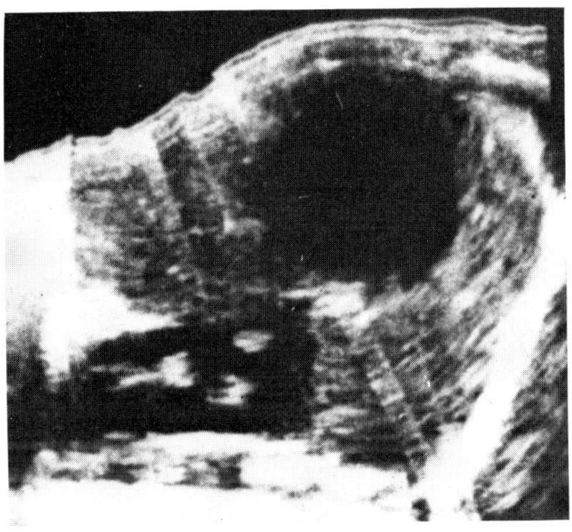

Fig. 13.9. *Amebic liver abscess*
Longitudinal scan through the right lobe of a liver with a 6 cm in diameter echo-poor lesion in the cranial part of the lobe, representing an amebic abscess.

**Pyogenic liver abscess** may be the cause of echo-poor lesions in the liver and clinically suspected in patients with a history of abdominal surgery, cholangitis and the like. Such a lesion may be punctured for diagnostic as well as therapeutic reasons. This is dealt with in chapter XVI.

**Hydatid disease** of the liver is an absolute contraindication for puncture, as this procedure may result in fatal anafylaxis or peritoneal dissemination. Ultrasonically, hydatids present either as ordinary cysts *(echinococcus hydatidosa)*, or as multilocular cysts *(echinococcus alveolaris)*. When hydatids become old they may be calcified. Suspicion of an echinococcus cysts is based upon geographical history, eosinophilia, pulmonary lesions, X-ray demonstration of calcifications in the liver, a positive Casoni skin reaction, serologic tests and possibly the demonstration of scolices (Fig. 13.10) in sputum. There is no medical therapy for this disease. Surgical treatment, i.e. extirpation in toto, offers the only hope of cure.

**Hepatic hemangiomas** when suspected should not be punctured. Fortunately, these tumors are rare. They are usually situated subcapsularly on the convexity of the right lobe of the liver. Clinically a vascular hum may be heard over the tumor and calcifications may be seen radiologically.

# References


Conn, H. O. and Yesmer, R.: A re-evaluation of needle biopsy in the diagnosis of metastatic cancer of the liver. *Annals Int. Med.* 53:59, 1963.

Rasmussen, S. N., Holm, H. H., Kristensen, J. K. and Barlebo, H.: Ultrasonically guided liver biopsy. *Br. Med. J.* 2:500, 1972.

Sherlock, S.: Diseases of the Liver and Biliary system, 5th ed. *Blackwell Scientific Publications,* Oxford 1975.

Söderström, N.: Fine Needle Aspiration Biopsy. *Almqvist and Wiksell,* Stockholm, 1966.

Triller, T.: Ultraschallgezielte abdominale Punktionen. *Radiologe* 19:173, 1979.

# CHAPTER XIV

# Ultrasonically guided percutaneous transhepatic portography

## Flemming Burcharth

Percutaneous transhepatic catheterization of the portal vein is a useful tool for visualization of the portal venous system in patients with liver cirrhosis and portal hypertension. The examination is also indicated in hepatomegaly, splenomegaly and in suspected tumors along the splenoportal pathway. By selective catheterization technique the method may also be used for obliteration of esophageal varices, and recently the method has been used to diagnose and localize endocrine pancreatic tumors.

## ANATOMY

In normal subjects the porta hepatis is placed about 3 cm to the right of the vertebral spine and about the width of a vertebral body anterior to the 12th thoracic vertebra. Accordingly the right branch of the portal vein should be entered by a puncture instrument introduced in the 9th intercostal space in the midaxillary line to a depth of 10–14 cm in the frontal plane. However, in cirrhosis of the liver there is often a marked deformation of normal anatomy, and the location of the porta hepatis may be several cm off the mark. In subjects without portal hypertension catheterization of the portal system is often only possible through puncture of a main portal branch in the porta hepatis.

## TECHNIQUE

Using landmarks of surface anatomy and fluoroscopy only, successful puncture may necessitate several attempts and depends on the investigator's tenacity. To improve the success rate of portal vein puncture, the exact position of the porta hepatis can be determined by ultrasonic scanning.

A commercially available static or dynamic scanner may be used. Transverse and longitudinal scans are recorded through the liver. The portal vein is seen at the porta hepatis as a transsonic

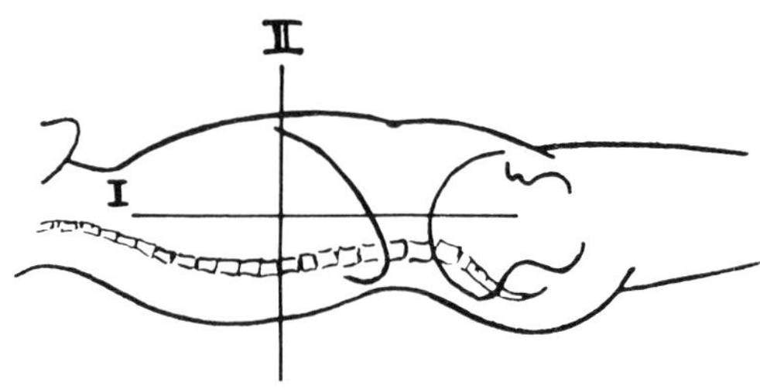

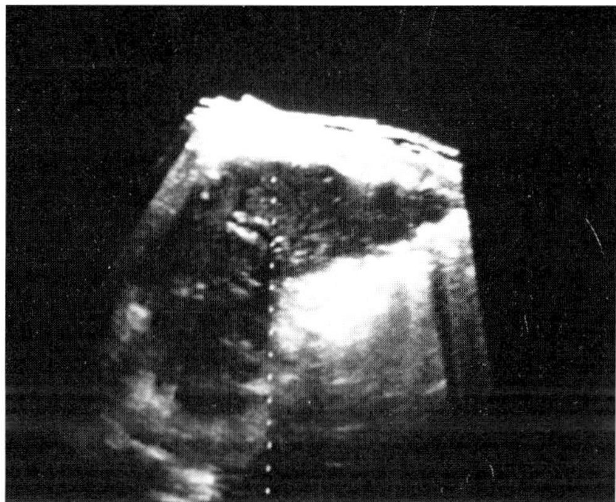

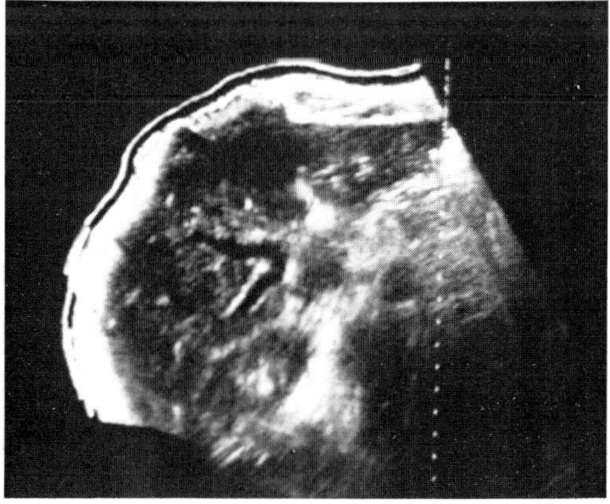

Fig. 14.1. The puncture site in percutaneous transhepatic porta catheterization, and examples of longitudinal (I) and transverse (II) liver scans used for localization of the porta hepatis. Branching of the right portal vein is seen.

structure with a well-defined wall producing strong echoes (Fig. 14.1). The division into right and left branches is often demonstrated, and the whole of the extrahepatic course of the portal and splenic veins can be assessed as totally or partially obstructed, normal or dilated. Dilated bile ducts and hepatic veins can be differentiated from intrahepatic portal veins since they are arranged differently within the liver and with a less defined wall.

From the ultrasonic scan a suitable point for puncture can be determined and marked on the patient (Fig. 14.1), and the distance from this point to the porta hepatis (right portal branch) is measured in the frontal plane.

The puncture and catheterization procedure is carried out in local analgesia and during fluoroscopic control with a soft polyethylene catheter provided with a steel mandrin (Fig. 14.2) as previously published by the author.

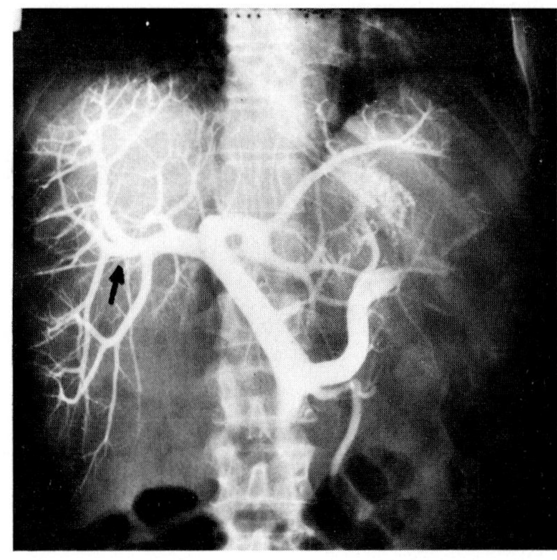

Fig. 14.2. Percutaneous transhepatic portogram from a patient with cirrhosis of the liver. The catheter enters the right portal vein 3–4 cm from the porta hepatis (black arrow).

## RESULTS

The results from 32 patients with ultrasonically guided porta catheterization have been compared with 32 patients without preceding ultrasonic scanning (Table 1). The method improved the puncture success rate from 80 to 97% ($P < 0.05$, Fisher's exact test) and reduced the number of puncture attempts before successful catheterization from an average of 5.1 to 2.1 ($P < 0.01$, Mann-Whitney test). The position of the porta hepatis determined by ultrasonic scanning was compared with the position determined from the portograms. In five cases deviations from 1 to 3 cm were recorded, in the other cases the agreement was complete.

Table 14.1. *Percutaneous transhepatic portography in 64 patients with and without preceding determination of the site of the porta hepatis by ultrasonic scanning*

| | Guided by ultrasonic scanning | | Without ultrasonic scanning | |
|---|---|---|---|---|
| | No. of patients | Average number of puncture attempts | No. of patients | Average number of puncture attempts |
| Successful examination | 31 | 2.1 | 25 | 5.1 |
| Unsuccessful examination | 1 | – | 7 | – |
| Total | 32 | | 32 | |

# References


Burcharth, F. and Rasmussen, S. N.: Localization of the porta hepatis by ultrasonic scanning prior to percutaneous transhepatic portography. *Br. J. Radiol.* 47:598, 1974.

Burcharth, F.: Percutaneous transhepatic portography. Technique and application. *Am. J. Roentgenol.* 132:177, 1979.

Filly, R. A. and Laing, F. C.: Anatomic variation of portal venous anatomy in the porta hepatis: Ultrasonographic evaluation. *J. Clin. Ultrasound* 6:83, 1978.

Hjortsjö, C.-H.: The topography of the intrahepatic duct systems. *Acta Anat.* (Basel) 11:599, 1950.

Webb, L. J., Berger, L. A. and Sherlock, S.: Grey-scale ultrasonography of portal vein. *Lancet* II, 675, 1977.

# CHAPTER XV

# Puncture of retroperitoneal, gastrointestinal and gynecological mass lesions

Jens Gammelgaard, Poul Hjortkær Pedersen and Ole Boll Henriksen

## RETROPERITONEAL MASS LESIONS

Apart from many of the abdominal viscera such as the pancreas, duodenum, colon, kidneys and great vessels which are located partly in the retroperitoneal space, the retroperitoneum is merely a space consisting of a layer of fat and connective tissue with lymph nodes and traversed by nerves and vessels.

Retroperitoneal mass lesions may be *primary retroperitoneal tumors,* like fibromas or sarcomas, or *secondary retroperitoneal tumors,* enlarged retroperitoneal lymph nodes, due to either generalized disease of the lymphatic system, or metastases from a malignant neoplasm.

The possible retroperitoneal origin of a mass lesion may be suggested ultrasonically from a well-circumscribed mass, possibly in close relation to the aorta and the inferior vena cava, separated from the surrounding organs, and not infrequently displacing or compressing the vein or even the aorta (Fig. 15.1).

Ultrasonically it is not possible to distinquish between a benign and a malignant retroperitoneal mass lesion. Fine needle aspiration biopsy has proven a useful and important tool in the diagnosis of retroperitoneal lesions. Ultrasonic scanning and biopsy is performed with the patient in the supine position. Intestinal gas may be an obstacle to a satisfactory and sufficient examination and it may be advantageous to repeat the examination with the patient in the fasting state. Biopsy of a retroperitoneal lesion requires no specific precautions. A guide needle is inserted only through the abdominal wall and a fine needle is introduced via the guide needle into the lesion. Usually the fine needle has to traverse the gastrointestinal tract, which can be done without risk.

It is a characteristic finding that retroperitoneal

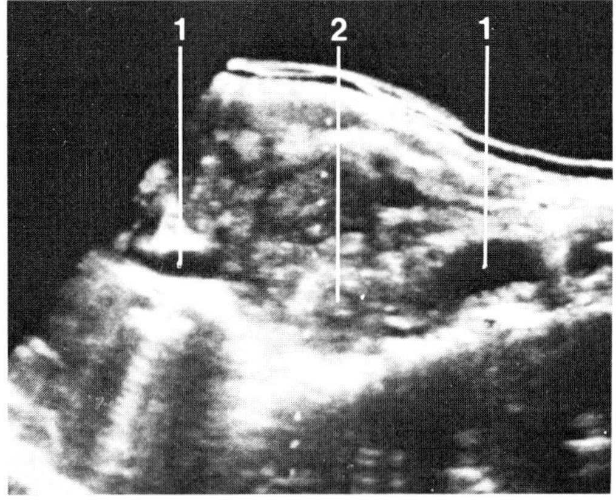


Fig. 15.1. *Retroperitoneal mass lesion*
Longitudinal scan through upper abdomen, near the midline. 1. Compressed inferior vena cava, 2. Retroperitoneal tumor.

masses are very firm to penetrate, and that aspirated material from a macroscopic point of view is very tissue poor.

In an 18-month period, 26 suspected retroperitoneal mass lesions have been subjected to fine needle aspiration biopsy (Table 15.1). Eighteen turned out to be malignant tumors, and eight were benign or no tumor at all. Thirteen malignant tumors were verified at autopsy or surgery and five on the basis of compelling clinical evidence. In two patients the malignant tumor was a primary malignant lymphoma, in one a huge carcinoma of the left adrenal. In 15 cases enlarged metastatic lymph nodes were secondary to carcinomas of the testis (four), kidney (four), colon (four), bladder (two) and pancreas (one), respectively. In the 18 patients with a malignant retroperitoneal tumor, malignant cells were aspirated from 14. In all 14 cases tumor cells were obtained on the first biopsy attempt, and easily recognizable microscopically

Tabel 15.1. *Retroperitoneal mass lesions*
The results of ultrasonically guided fine needle aspiration biopsy of 26 suspected retroperitoneal mass lesions.

|  |  | Malig-<br>nant<br>cells | No malig-<br>nant<br>cells | Insuf-<br>ficient<br>material |
|---|---|---|---|---|
| Malignant | 18 | 14 | 1 | 3 |
| Benign | 8 | 0 | 8 | 0 |
| Total | 26 | 14 | 9 | 3 |

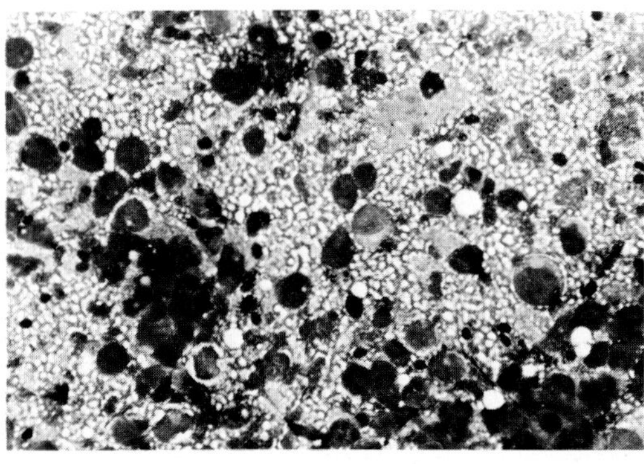

Fig. 15.4. *Cytology: Metastasis from seminoma of the testis*
Highly cellular material with rather monotonous picture of medium-sized immature cells having moderate amounts of pale, often ill-defined cytoplasm, fairly pale, large nuclei with large nucleoli. (× 300).

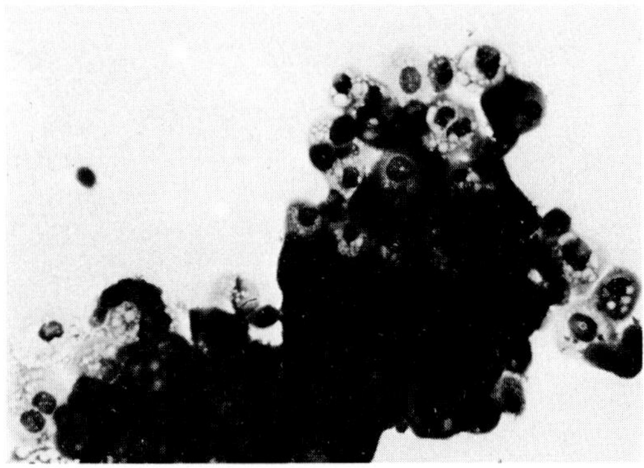

Fig. 15.2. *Cytology: Metastasis from renal carcinoma*
Irregular sheet of epithelial cells with some degree of nuclear size variation and hyperchromasia. Cytoplasm rather abundant and vacuolated. (× 300).

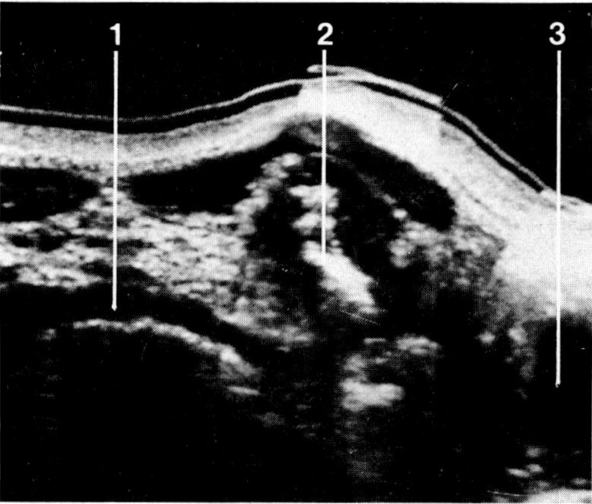


Fig. 15.5. *Solid tumor in the sigmoid*
Longitudinal scan through lower abdomen. 1. Aorta, 2. Solid tumor in the sigmoid, 3. Bladder.

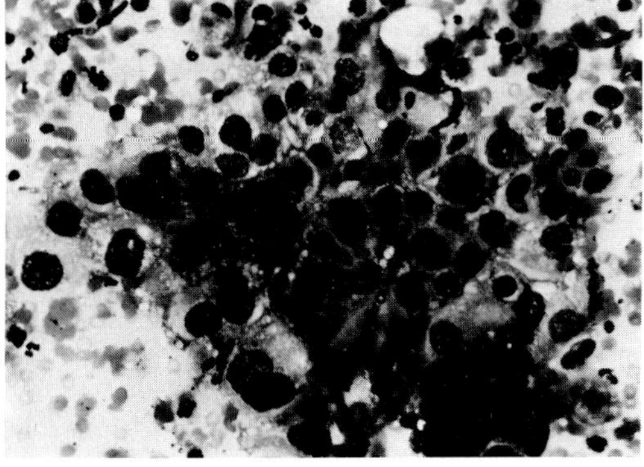

Fig. 15.3. *Cytology: Metastasis from anaplastic bladder carcinoma*
Sheet of highly polymorphous epithelial cells with hyperchromatic nuclei of varying size and varying amounts of ill-defined pale cytoplasm. (× 300).

(Figs. 15.2, 15.3, 15.4 and 15.5). In one patient no malignant cells were obtained and histological examination of the surgically removed tumor proved it to be completely necrotic, containing no identifiable tumor cells. In three cases the aspirated material was insufficient for a conclusive cytologic diagnosis. There were no false positive biopsies.

## GASTROINTESTINAL MASS LESIONS

It has been generally accepted that ultrasound scanning is of no importance in the evaluation of



Retroperitoneal, gastrointestinal and gynecological mass lesions

tumors of the GI tract. However, this has turned out to be only a qualified truth.

A gastrointestinal tumor has a characteristic ultrasonic appearance with a rounded rather well-circumscribed, echo-poor area, with strong echoes centrally from the lumen of the organ (Fig. 15.5) Another characteristic is that the scanning is impeded by bowel gas. It may be helpful to press the transducer against the abdominal wall to displace the gas.

When a mass lesion with the above-mentioned characteristics has been disclosed, a fine needle biopsy should be considered.

The ultrasonic scanning and the biopsy are performed with the patient in the supine position and no special precaution has to be taken. A guide needle is introduced only through the abdominal wall and a fine needle is advanced via the guide needle into the tumor.

In a personal investigation during an 8-month period, ultrasound scanning revealed a picture suspicious of a GI tract tumor in 16 patients. In seven patients the tumor was primarily discovered at the ultrasound scanning, in five by some X-ray procedure, at endoscopy in two, and at surgery and gynecological examination in one case, respectively. Four tumors were located in the stomach, nine in the large bowel, and three in the rectum. In all 16 patients fine needle aspiration biopsy was performed. No complications to the biopsy were discovered.

Fourteen of the 16 suspected mass lesions were verfified at autopsy or surgery to be malignant tumors (Table 15.2).

In only one patient with a malignant tumor no malignant cells were obtained by biopsy. In two patients with peridiverticulitis of the sigmoid, no

Tabel 15.2. *Gastrointestinal mass lesions*
The results of ultrasonically guided fine needle aspiration biopsy of 16 suspected gastrointestinal mass lesions.

|  |  | Malignant cells | No malignant cells | Insufficient material |
|---|---|---|---|---|
| Malignant | 14 | 13 | 1 | 0 |
| Benign | 2 | 0 | 2 | 0 |
| Total | 16 | 13 | 3 | 0 |

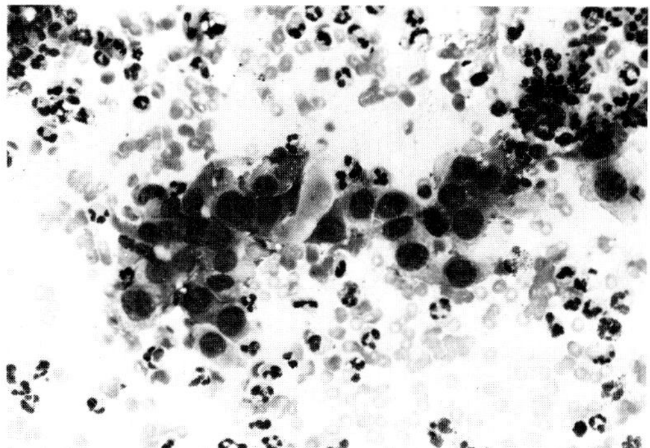

Fig. 15.6. *Cytology: Adenocarcinoma of the colon* Groups of epithelial cells with variation in cell and nuclear size and hyperchromatic nuclei often with large nucleoli. Cell shape irregular often elongated. (× 300).

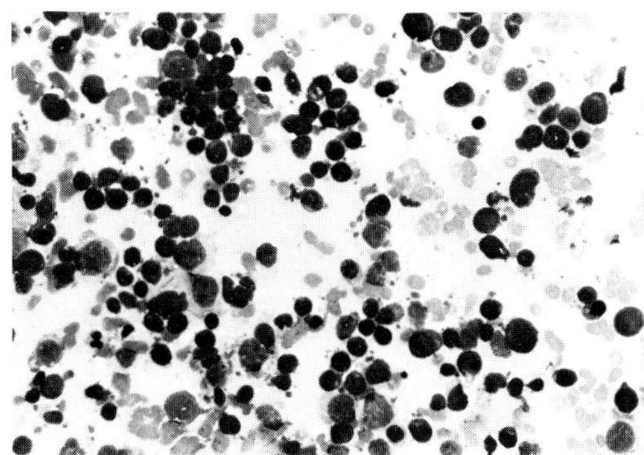

Fig. 15.7. *Cytology: Malignant lymphoma of the stomach* No clearly epithelial cells but numerous lymphocytic cells with a varying differentiation hyperchromatic sometimes irregular nuclei often containing nucleoli and fairly abundant cytoplasm. Many small lymphocytes are also seen. (× 300).

malignant cells were obtained. In all cases the aspirated material was sufficient for a conclusive cytologic diagnosis (Figs. 15.6 and 15.7).

This investigation does not imply that ultrasound scanning is the examination of choice in the search for gastrointestinal tumors. It emphasizes, however, that whenever a mass lesion with these characteristics is demonstrated, a fine needle biopsy can in most cases verify the malignant nature of the tumor.

# GYNECOLOGICAL MASS LESIONS

By ultrasonic scanning it is possible to visualize gynecological tumors with a high degree of certainty (Figs. 15.8 and 15.9). However, it is generally accepted that the differential diagnosis between malignant and benign gynecological lesions is difficult and unsatisfactory when based on ultrasonic scanning alone.

Meire et al. investigated the possibility of a distinction of benign from malignant ovarian cysts by ultrasound. They used the following parameters,

1. size of lesion,
2. unilocular,
3. multilocular,
4. presence of thin septa (less than 3 mm),
5. presence of thick septa (greater than 3 mm),
6. presence of solid nodules,
7. evidence of invasion of capsule,
8. evidence of fixation of mass.

The two last-mentioned criteria were found to be very subjective and unreliable, but using the first-mentioned six criteria an accuracy of 91% was obtained. Suspected of malignancy were large multiloculated cysts with thin septa and nodules or multiloculated cysts with thick septa with or without nodules.

Ultrasound scanning may restrict the number of other preoperative examinations. This is especially the case when a mobile, unilocular cyst without nodules is demonstrated.

Fine needle puncture has been performed in solid and cystic gynecological mass lesions for many years. The technique has mostly been that described by Franzén using a fine needle (0.6 mm) mounted on a 10 ml syringe. The needle was previously inserted into the cystic or solid tumor guided by palpation.

In the literature the accuracy of the cytological diagnoses in ovarian tumors varies considerably. Kjellgren et al. had 7.7% and Jensen et al. 16% false diagnoses. The material obviously consisted of benign as well as malignant lesions and the percentages stated were "over-all accuracies".

From Jensen et al.'s work the number of false negatives can be calculated to be 38%. The predictive value of a negative finding is therefore quite unsatisfactory in the evaluation of patients with gynecological mass lesions. A patient in the "cancer age" who presents with a gynecological mass lesion has to be operated upon despite a negative cytological diagnosis.

Even though the blind biopsies can now be substituted by ultrasonically guided fine needle aspiration biopsies from suspicious areas of the tumor,

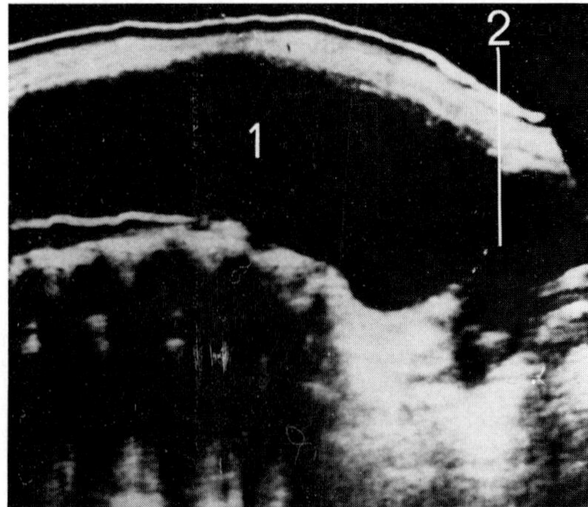

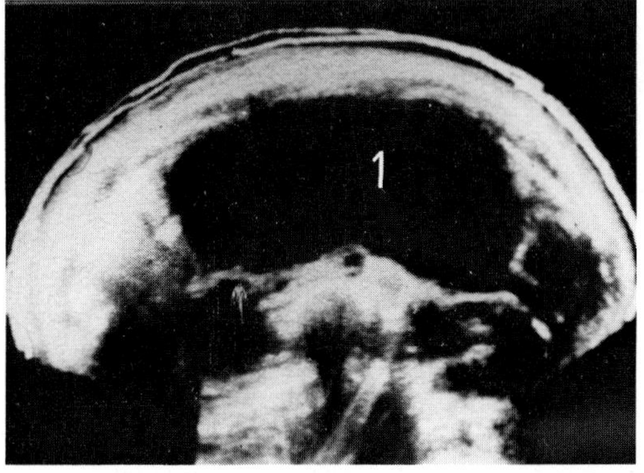

Fig. 15.8. *Large monoloculated ovarian cyst*
Above, longitudinal section, below, transverse section.
1. Cyst, 2. Urinary bladder.

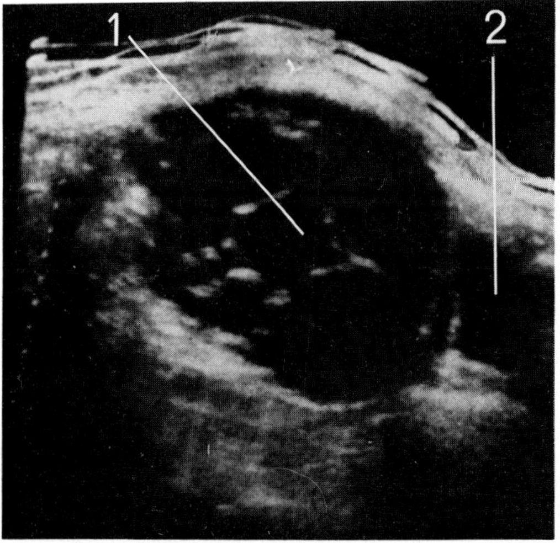

Fig. 15.9. *Multiloculated ovarian cyst*
1. Cyst, 2. Urinary bladder.

     Retroperitoneal, gastrointestinal and gynecological mass lesions

it is not likely that the number of false negatives can be reduced sufficiently to make the method clinically valuable. An obvious pitfall is presented by the multiloculated cyst in which it is difficult to obtain material from all compartments. Malignant transformation, which may occur in the smallest compartment, may therefore be difficult to exclude.

Since a biopsy will have no consequence in these patients who will be operated upon in any case, it does not seem reasonable to perform biopsies even though complications are rare (2.9% — mainly fever and signs of intraabdominal bleeding — in the material of Jensen et al.).

Much effort has been made to try to find other parameters which might improve the diagnostic value of punctures. Tropé et al. determined the DNA activity and the presence of fibrin/fibrinogen degradation products (FDP) in the ovarian cystic fluid or ascites and found that in 90% of the cases an increased DNA synthesis and the presence of FDP indicated malignancy.

A serious argument against the use of puncture of suspected malignant gynecological lesions is the possibility that cancer cells leak into the peritoneal cavity. This may also interfere with the staging of ovarian carcinoma advocated by the International Federation of Gynecology and Obstetrics (FIGO) in 1970. This staging method includes substages with free cancer cells in the peritoneal cavity. It is not known with certainty , however, if this is of prognostic importance in stages I and II of the disease. Since penetration of the tumor capsule by needle puncture with possible leaking of tumor cells into the peritoneal cavity may complicate the problem, preoperative puncture is at present avoided in patients with suspected ovarian cancer.

However, ultrasonically guided puncture is valuable in patients with suspected, inoperable malignant disease who are unfit for surgery. A diagnosis can be established without a potentially risky laparotomy and chemotherapy can be initiated. Furthermore suspected focal liver lesions may be punctured and if liver metastases are present, an operation may be omitted and chemotherapy started.

Cystic ovarian masses in young women are seldom malignant. In these patients ultrasonically guided puncture may have great possibilities in the future since retention cysts (follicular or luteal) may disappear after puncture. While these patients may be spared an operation, the patients with "real" neoplasms such as serous cysts, pseudomucinous cysts and dermoid cysts must go to surgery since malignancy may develop in these tumors.

A method which, based on the determination of some specific components in the cyst fluid, could differentiate between retention cysts and real neoplasms would therefore be most valuable.

Other space-occupying lesions related to gynecology lend themselves to ultrasonically guided puncture: Lymphomas after radical hysterectomy, hematomas after gynecological operations, abscesses in the true pelvis and peritoneal cysts caused by adhesions or infections.

# References


Berkowitz, R. S., Leavitt, T. and Knapp, R. C.: Ultrasound-directed percutaneous aspiration biopsy of periaortic lymph nodes in recurrence of cervical carcinoma. *Am. J. Obstet. Gynecol.,* 131:906, 1978.

Doust, B.: The use of ultrasound in the diagnosis of gastroenterological disease. *Gastroenterol.* 70:602, 1976.

Frank, Von W. B., Menges, V. and Klein, M.: Die Ultraschalldiagnostik bei wandinfiltrativen Prozessen des Intestinaltraktes. *Fortschr. Roentgenstr.* 129:90, 1978.

Franzén, S.: Studier över värdet av punktionscytologi vid diagnostik av tumor sjukdomar (thesis). *Edilin-Malm,* Stockholm, 1968.

Jensen, H. K., Gram, N. C. and Francis, D.: Finnålspunktur som diagnostisk hjælpemiddel ved gynækologiske tumorer. *Ugeskr. Læg.* 136:586, 1974.

Kjellgren, O., Ångström, T., Bergman, F. and Wiklund, D.–E.: Fine-needle aspiration biopsy in diagnosis and classification of ovarian carcinoma. *Cancer* 28:967, 1971.

Leopold, G. R. and Asher, M. W.: Diagnosis of extraorgan retroperitoneal space lesions by B-scan ultrasonography. *Radiol.* 103:133, 1972.

Lutz, H. Th. and Petzoldt, R.: Ultrasonic patterns of space occupying lesions of the stomach and the intestine. *Ultrasound Med. Biol.* 2:129, 1976.

Mascatello, V. J., Carrera, G. F., Teele, R. L., Berger, M., Holm, H. H. and Smith, E. H.: The ultrasonic demonstration of gastric lesions. *J. Clin. Ultrasound* 5:383, 1977.

Meire, H. B., Farrant, P. and Guha, T.: Distinction of benign from malignant ovarian cysts by ultrasound. *Br. J. Obstet. Gynecol.* 85:893, 1978.

Schwerk, Von W. B. and Braun, B.: Ultraschalldiagnostik gastrointestinaler Tumoren. *Zeitschr. Gastroenterol.* 16:431, 1978.

Tropé, C., Persson, P. H. and Svanberg, L.: Preoperative diagnosis of malignancy of ovarian cysts. Paper presented at XX Nordic Congress of Obstetrics and Gynecology. Abstract No. 33.

Walls, W. J.: The evaluation of malignant gastric neoplasm by ultrasonic B scanning. *Radiol.* 119:159, 1976.

Weidenhiller, S., Lutz, H. Th. and Petzoldt, R.: Ultraschallgezielte Feinnadelpunktion von abdominalen und retroperitonealen Tumoren. *Med. Klin.:* 70:973, 1975.

# CHAPTER XVI

# Puncture of intraabdominal fluid collections

Orla Als

The non-operative verification or exclusion of an intraabdominal fluid collection is difficult. Clinical examination is in most cases unable to demonstrate such a collection unless it has reached a considerable size or is located superficially. Conventional radiology is not very useful either unless the abscess displaces adjacent organs or if gas has developed inside the abscess cavity. The more recently introduced gallium scanning is time consuming, and it is not quite specific in the differentiation between abscesses and tumors.

Several publications have confirmed that ultrasonic scanning of the abdomen is a most valuable tool in the diagnostic armamentarium when an intraabdominal fluid collection is suspected. The accuracy of the method seems in experienced hands to exceed 90%. However, in the majority of cases it is not possible, based on the ultrasonic findings alone, to determine the nature of the fluid in a localized, echo-free or echo-poor lesion. Especially abscesses and hematomas are identical in echo configuration.

If an intraabdominal fluid collection is present, an ultrasonically guided percutaneous puncture is often indicated in order to determine the nature of the fluid.

## PROCEDURE

When a fluid-filled lesion has been disclosed, the optimum site, direction and depth for the puncture are determined. The skin is sterilized, local anesthetic applied and the puncture performed via a static or dynamic puncture transducer as described in chapter IV. A cannula with an outer diameter of 1.2 mm is always used.

When the needle has been introduced to the predetermined depth, the lesion is emptied by aspiration with a sterile syringe or automatic suction. In a few cases when fluid can not be aspirated, it is often an advantage to inject and aspirate a small amount of saline in order to get sufficient material for relevant examinations.

Using a conventional static scanner it is useful to watch the A-scope because in this mode the needle tip is visualized as a sharp echo spike inside the lesion, and the position of the needle can be adjusted during the aspiration. Also in this mode the echo-free lesion will be seen to disappear gradually with emptying. The use of a dynamic scanner will provide the same information (Fig. 16.1).

## Handling of the aspirated material

Material aspirated from a localized, intraabdominal fluid collection should always be sent to the

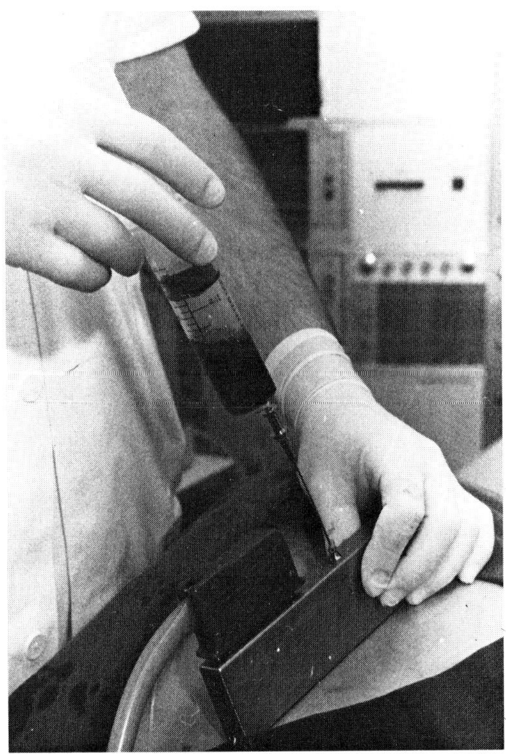

Fig. 16.1. *Ultrasonically guided fluid aspiration*
The puncture is in this case performed through a dynamic (linear array) puncture transducer.

bacteriologist for aerobic as well as anaerobic cultures (see chapter VII). The bacteriologist should be provided with relevant clinical information, including possible antibiotic treatment. When malignancy cannot be ruled out, fluid should also be examined cytologically. When more specific types of fluid are suspected, biochemical tests may be applied, e.g. creatinine in suspected urinomas, protein in suspected seromas or lymphoceles and amylase in suspected pancreatic pseudocysts.

## DIAGNOSTIC PUNCTURE

In a series of 72 patients ultrasonically guided aspirations of localized intraabdominal fluid collections were performed for diagnostic purposes. The size of these collections varied from a few ml to more than 2000 ml; the locations were numerous (Table 16.1). The nature of the fluid is indicated in Table 16.2.

Table 16.1.

| | |
|---|---|
| Subphrenic | 10 |
| Intrahepatic | 3 |
| Subhepatic | 9 |
| Perirenal | 7 |
| Adjacent renal grafts | 10 |
| Lower quadrants | 10 |
| True pelvic | 15 |
| Interintestinal | 8 |
| Total | 72 |

Localization of intraabdominal fluid collection – punctures for diagnostic purpose.

Table 16.2.

| | |
|---|---|
| Pus | 38 |
| Blood | 15 |
| Ascitic fluid | 7 |
| Lymph | 7 |
| Undefined | 2 |
| No fluid | 3 |
| Total | 72 |

Character of aspirated fluid.

In 69 cases material for further examination was aspirated, while this was not possible in three cases. In two of these cases subsequent surgery revealed an abscess at the ultrasonically predicted subhepatic location. The reason for these failures is uncertain. In the third case venous blood was aspirated in an attempt to puncture a $3 \times 3 \times 4$ cm echo-poor lesion, located subhepatically anterior to the inferior vena cava. The procedure was then stopped. The final diagnosis is uncertain in this case since exploratory laparotomy was not indicated.

If possible, puncture through the liver is avoided. In many cases part of the gastrointestinal tract has been penetrated. In no case complications related to the procedure were registered.

In 38 cases pus was aspirated with cultures demonstrating bacterial growth in 29 cases.

## THERAPEUTIC PUNCTURE

Laparotomy with large tube drainage has always been the established treatment of an intraabdominal abscess.

Recently there have been reported a few cases where intraabdominal abscesses have been cured by means of an ultrasonically guided puncture with subsequent emptying of the cavity or Seldinger catheterization, both combined with instillation of antibiotics.

When an intraabdominal abscess has been diagnosed by ultrasonic scanning and subsequent puncture, the following procedure has been used:
1. The abscess is aspirated completely.
2. The cavity is irrigated with saline several times, until the returning fluid is clear.
3. An antibiotic combination with broad spectrum and low toxicity is injected into the abscess cavity (ampicillin 1 g + cephaloridin 1 g in 10 ml $H_2O$).
4. A control scanning is performed after a few days and if a fluid collection is still present the procedure is repeated.
5. In some cases where puncture of organs in front of the abscess can be excluded, a polyethylene catheter with an outer diameter of 2 mm is introduced by the Seldinger technique and left in place for drainage and subsequent irrigations.

A series of 12 patients with intraabdominal



Intraabdominal fluid collections

abscesses have been treated according to the above principles (Table 16.3). The localization is shown in Table 16.4.

The four abscesses in the hepatic region were treated with catheterization combined with antibiotics. Three were cured. One had a recurrence 9 days after removal of the catheter; eight were treated with aspiration and antibiotics; five of these were cured.

One was unfortunately operated upon the day after puncture and antibiotic instillation. The operation was probably not necessary since the contents were found to be sterile at the time of surgery whereas the material aspirated the day before showed growth of hemolytic streptococci.

One periappendiceal abscess was caused by a large perforation of the colon and a hemicolectomi was necessary.

One perforated spontaneously to the rectum 10 days after puncture.

Blood cultures before and after puncture have been performed, and bacteriemia induced by puncture was never seen.

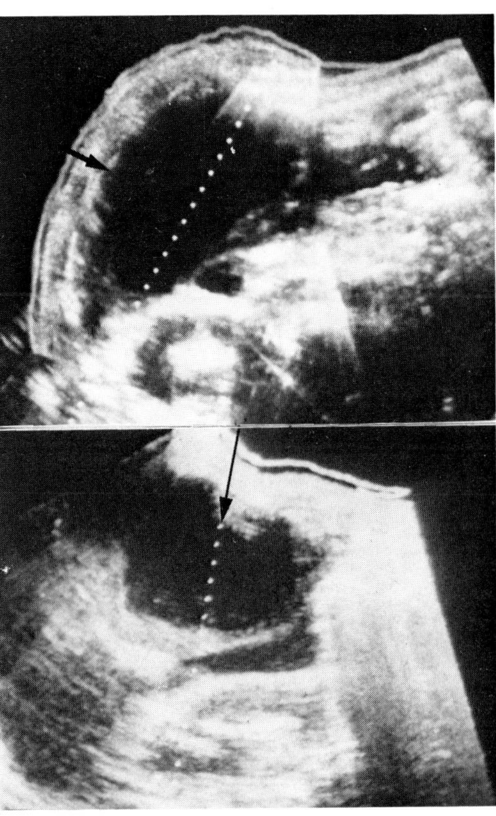

Fig. 16.2. *Large liver abscess*
Above, transverse scan, below, longitudinal scan. A large echo-free space representing an abscess is seen in the right lobe of the liver. Postero-medially is seen the gall bladder and the right kidney.

Table 16.3.

*12 abscesses treated with aspiration and antibiotics*

|            |    | Cured | Not cured |
|------------|----|-------|-----------|
| + catheter | 4  | 3     | 1         |
| − catheter | 8  | 5     | 3         |
| Total      | 12 | 8     | 4         |

Table 16.4.

| Subhepatic     | 2  |
|----------------|----|
| Intrahepatic   | 2  |
| Retroperitoneal| 1  |
| Pelvic         | 1  |
| Periappendiceal| 6  |
| Total          | 12 |

Localization of abscesses – treated by puncture and antibiotics locally.

## Case report

A 38-year-old male had upper abdominal pain and spiking fever for 12 days.

The ultrasound scan showed a large echo-poor area inside the right lobe of the liver (Fig. 16.2). Ultrasonically guided puncture revealed 450 ml pus, containing non hemolytic streptococci. Antibiotics were instilled. The following day the temperature was normal and the patient felt quite well. Follow-up scanning with puncture 4 days later revealed a lesion containing 80 ml of fluid, as did scanning with puncture 3 weeks later. At this time Seldinger catheterization of the lesion was performed. The output diminished successively, and it is remarkable that after the second aspiration the fluid was sterile. Ultrasound scan 3 months later was almost normal (Fig. 16.3).

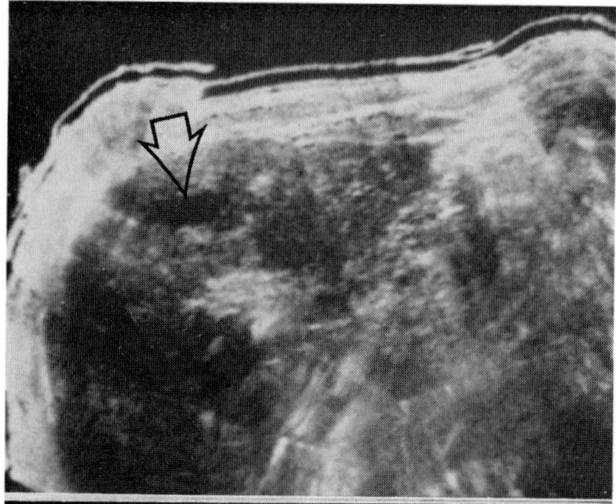

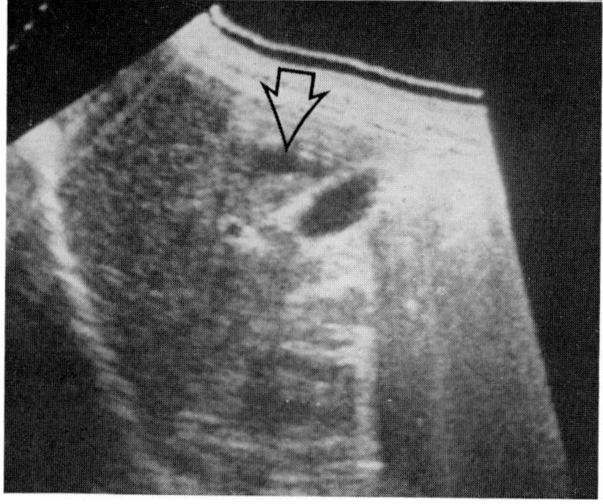

Fig. 16.3. *Control scanning of liver abscess*
Above, transverse scan, below, longitudinal scan.
The scans are obtained 3 months after puncture of the
liver abscess seen in Fig. 16.2. The scans are almost
normal. Only a small homogeneous area cephalad to the
gall bladder remains (arrow marked).

When an ultrasonic scanning reveals a localized intraabdominal fluid collection, an ultrasonically guided percutaneous puncture gives important diagnostic information. The procedure is simple, rapid, and effective to determine the exact nature of the fluid and it is without risk and almost without discomfort to the patient. A superfluous operation may be avoided in patients where the aspiration reveals a hematoma, ascitic fluid, etc.

The preliminary results by treating intraabdominal abscesses by ultrasonically guided aspiration combined with antibiotics locally in the cavity and perhaps Seldinger catheterization seem promising, but more experience is obviously needed.

No complications were registered.

# References


Conrad, M. R., Sanders, R. C. and Mascardo, A.: Perinephric abscess aspiration using ultrasound guidance. *Am. J. Roentgenol.* 128:464, 1977.

Doust, B. D., Quiroz, F. and Steward, J. M.: Ultrasonic distinction of abscesses from other intraabdominal fluid collections. *Radiol.* 125: 213, 1977.

Grønvall, J., Grønvall, S. and Hegedüs, V.: Ultrasound-guided drainage of fluid-containing masses using angiographic catheterization techniques. *Am. J. Roentgenol.* 129:997, 1977.

Holm, H. H., Pedersen, J. F., Kristensen, J. K., Rasmussen, S. N., Hancke, S. and Jensen, F.: Ultrasonically guided percutaneous puncture. *Radiol. Clin. North Am.* 13:493, 1975.

Jensen, F. and Pedersen, J. F.: The value of ultrasonic scanning in the diagnosis of intraabdominal abscesses and hematomas. *Surg. Gynecol. Obstet.* 139:326, 1974.

Lavender, J. P., Barker, J. R. and Chaudhri, M. A.: Gallium-67 citrate scanning in neoplastic and inflammatory lesions. *Br. J. Radiol.* 44:361, 1977.

Maklad, N. F., Doust, B. D. and Baum, J. K.: Ultrasonic diagnosis of postoperative intraabdominal abscesses. *Radiol.* 113:417, 1974.

Pedersen, J. F., Hancke, S. and Kristensen, J. K.: Renal Carbuncle: antibiotic therapy governed by ultrasonically guided aspiration. *J. Urol.* 109:777, 1973.

Smith, E. H. and Bartrum, R. S.: Ultrasonically guided percutaneous aspiration of abscesses. *Am. J. Roentgenol. Radium Ther. Nucl. Med.* 122:308, 1974.

Taylor, K. J. W., Wasson, J., DeGraaff, C., Rosenfield, A. T. and Andriole, V. T.: Accuracy of grey-scale ultrasound diagnosis of abdominal and pelvic abscesses in 220 patients. *Lancet* 1:83, 1978.

# CHAPTER XVII

# Amniocentesis in early pregnancy

Jens Bang and John Philip

Since Bevis demonstrated the value of examination of the amniotic fluid for assessment of erythoblastosis in the third trimester, indications for amniocentesis have been greatly extended. In the third trimester amniocentesis is now done for several reasons, such as assessment of fetal maturity and determination of biochemical parameters in erythroblastosis.

## INDICATIONS

Also in the second trimester amniocentesis is now widely used for genetic diagnosis. Chromosomal disorders may be diagnosed by cytogenetic examination of fetal cells from the amniotic fluid. Inborn errors of metabolism may be diagnosed by studies of fetal cells or in a few cases by examination of amniotic fluid.

Neural tube defects may be revealed by the study of the alfa-fetoprotein content of the amniotic fluid. Fetal sex may be determined in families with X-linked diseases.

The number of second trimester amniocenteses is growing rapidly. The number of prenatal genetic diagnoses carried out has been limited by lack of funds in most countries. In Denmark, however, a special appropriation was given in October 1978 to allow, that 1) every pregnant woman 35 years or more, 2) pregnant women who have previously borne a child with a chromosome anomaly, and 3) families in whom either the pregnant woman or her husband has a translocation or another chromosomal aberration, should be offered genetic counselling and a prenatal diagnosis, if they wish; 3000–4000 second trimester amniocenteses are estimated necessary for these purposes per year in Denmark.

## METHOD

Amniocentesis should be carried out under ultrasound guidance, because of higher success rates: In a Canadian collaborative study by Simpson et al., the success rates by first amniocentesis improved from 76% to 86% after placental localization by ultrasound, and Crandon & Peel showed an increase in the success rate of amniocentesis from 80 to 99,6% after the introduction of ultrasound guidance. The incidence of blood contamination in the amniotic fluid was similarly reduced from 43.5 til 17.6%.

Since the beginning of the 1970s we have used an ultrasonic puncture transducer allowing amniocentesis under simultaneous visual ultrasound guidance. The degree of contraction of the uterus and the position of the fetus can be seen during the procedure.

If this visualization technique cannot be used, it is of great importance to do the amniocentesis immediately after the ultrasonic scanning, so that alterations of the uterine contraction do not take place.

In order to localize the placenta, to estimate the length of the gestation and the number of fetuses, and to secure fetal heart movement, ultrasound scanning is first carried out. The standard transducer is then exchanged with the puncture transducer, which has been sterilized. The skin is swabbed with iodine. Local anesthesia is never used (most patients find that the puncture hurts less than the taking of a blood sample).

The puncture transducer is placed directly over an area of free fluid and the needle (1.2 mm/ 14 cm) is introduced into the cavity. The needle is visualized on the scanning picture as well as on the A-presentation. 15 ml of amniotic fluid are routinely aspirated into a syringe and transported to the cytogenetic laboratory in the same syringe.

In cases of twins we have developed a special technique. After the aspiration of fluid from one gestational sac, 2 ml of Congo red 1.5% are injected into the amniotic cavity. A new puncture near the second fetus is made. If the amniotic fluid removed is of normal color, samples from both cavities have been obtained.

# RESULTS

Table 17.1 demonstrates the outcome of the first 1177 pregnancies investigated by amniocentesis. All cases have been followed up after delivery. Of all 1183 infants, 1118 (94.5%) were born alive: 1039 (87.8%) weighed over 2500 g, and 79 (6.7%) under 2500 g. Twenty-six terminations were performed, 13 because of chromosomal abnormalities, the rest because of raised alfa-fetoprotein concentration, rubella infection, male fetuses in families with X-linked diseases, maternal diabetes, and adrenogenital syndrome. In one of the four cases of twins not detected by ultrasound before amniocentesis, a liveborn infant with Downs syndrome was delivered, and in one case where the cells did not grow a mongoloid child was later born. Otherwise no visible malformations caused by cromosome abnormalities were found. No damage caused by the amniocentesis was recorded after delivery.

Twenty-eight pregnancies (2.4%) ended in spontaneous abortions (Table 17.2). Although amniocentesis was usually performed during or after the 16th week of gestation, in about one-quarter of the cases it was performed before. The earlier the amniocentesis is performed, the more likely is the mother to have spontaneous abortion independent of the amniocentesis. In three of the 28 cases (10.7%) repeated punctures were necessary owing to difficulties in obtaining fluid or in culturing cells. The overall incidence of repeated punctures in the series was 3% (see below). Only six of the spontaneous abortions occurred in women under 35 years of age (Table 17.2). The mean age of all 28 cases was 35 years, range 23–49.

Three of the 1177 women (0.3%) had their first symptom of abortion within 8 days after amniocentesis. Eight (0.7%) had their first symptom between 8 days and 3 weeks and 17 (1.4%) after 3 weeks. Eleven of the 28 women already had conditions associated with an increased risk of abortion. Eight others probably had such conditions. Risk factors noted in the series were bleeding, cervical insufficiency, hydrocephalus, twins, intrauterine device in situ, and abnormalities of the placenta. None of the fetuses aborted spontaneously had a chromosomal abnormality. Simpson et al. have shown that the risk of abortion increases

Table 17.1. *Outcome of 1177 pregnancies after amniocentesis*

| | Born alive | | Stillborn | Spontaneous abortions | Induced abortions | Total infants* |
|---|---|---|---|---|---|---|
| | > 2500 g | < 2500 g | | | | |
| No (%) of infants | 1039(87·8) | 79(6·7) | 11(0·9) | 28(2·4) | 26(2·2) | 1183(100·0) |

* Six cases were twin pregnancies

Table 17.2. *Indications for amniocentesis and incidences of spontaneous abortion*

| | Maternal age > 40 | Maternal age 35–39 | Other (maternal age < 35) | Total |
|---|---|---|---|---|
| No of amniocentesis | 256 | 469 | 454 | 1179* |
| No(%) of spontaneous abortions | 8(3·1) | 14(3·0) | 6(1·3) | 28(2·4) |

* Includes two cases in which twins were diagnosed before amniocentesis.



Amniocentesis in early pregnancy

when amniocentesis proves difficult to perform or needs to be repeated.

In our center immediate complications are few. Out of 1760 consecutive amniocenteses performed from March 1973 to February 1978, 42 (2.4%) produced macroscopically blood-stained fluid. In 32 cases (1,8%) two punctures were made the same day, and in 19 (1.1%) a second puncture was made a week later. In the last two-thirds of the cases, when the obstetricians had gained optimum experience with the technique, only 1.5% of the samples contained macroscopic blood and 0.2% of the patients needed a second puncture a week later.

The incidence of fetal loss after amniocentesis may be assessed indirectly by comparison with figures for prematurity and abortions.

In our series the incidence of premature birth was 6.7% while for the whole of Denmark during 1976 it was 6% (Danmarks Statistik). Obel in Copenhagen and Shapiro et al. in New York who analyzed spontaneous abortion rates among women of various ages and of various periods of gestation, reported incidences among women not examined by amniocentesis similar to that found in our series. Shapiro found 3.2% after the 15th week of gestation and Obel 2.7% in all ages.

Of the 28 women in our series who aborted spontaneously after amniocentesis, 11 were probably already at risk of aborting. Of the remainder, eight (0.7% of all mothers) had their first symptom of abortion within 3 weeks after the procedure. If a time interval of 3 weeks is considered to be a reasonable limit, these eight cases may have been causally associated with amniocentesis. Three women without risk factors associated with abortion had the first symptom within 1 week after the procedure. If this is regarded as a reasonable time limit, 0.25% of all mothers may have aborted as a result of amniocentesis.

Our findings suggest that amniocentesis in early pregnancy does entail a small risk of spontaneous abortion. Nevertheless, about 0.5% of newborn babies have chromosomal abnormalities. Confining amniocentesis to women over 35 results in only 20–30% of cases of Down's syndrome being detected before birth, as demonstrated by Mikkelsen et al.

The overall incidence of abortion after the 15th week of pregnancy and independent of maternal age is 2–2.5%. Our findings suggest that if all pregnant women undergo amniocentesis, the incidence will increase by 0.3 – 0.7%. This, however, must be weighed against the 70–80% of cases of Down's syndrome and even higher proportions of other genetic disorders that go unrecognized before birth.

# References


Bevis, D. C. A.: Composition of liquor amnii in haemolytic disease of newborn. *Lancet* 2:443, 1959.

Simpson, N. E., Dallairi, L., Miller, J. R., Siminovich, L., Hamerton, J. L., Miller, J. and Mckeen, C.: Prenatal diagnosis of genetic disease in Canada: report of a collaborative study. *Can. Med. Assoc. J.* 115:39, 1976.

Crandon, A. J. and Peel, K. R.: Amniocentesis with and without ultrasound guidance. *Br. J. Obstet. Gynecol.* 86:1, 1979.

Holm, J. H., Kristensen, J. K., Rasmussen, S. N., Nortehved, A., and Barlebo, H.: *Ultrasonics* 83:83, 1972.

Bang, J., and Northeved A.: A new ultrasonic method for transabdominal amniocentesis. *Am. J. Obstet. Gynecol.* 114, 599, 1972.

Bang, J., Nielsen, H., and Philip, J.: Prenatal karyotyping of twins by ultrasonically guided amniocentesis. *Am. J. Obstet. Gynecol.* 123: 695, 1975.

Philip, J., and Bang, J.: Outcome of pregnancy after amniocentesis for chromosome analysis. *Br. Med. J.* 2:1183, 1978.

Obel, E.: Risk of spontaneous abortion following legal abortion. To be published.

Shapiro, S., Jones, E. W., and Densen, P. M.: A life of pregnancy terminations and correlates of fetal loss. *Milbank Memorial Found Quartely.* 40:7, 1962.

Mikkelsen, M., Fischer, G., Stene, J., Stene, E., and Petersen, E.: Incidence study of Down's syndrom in Copenhagen, 1960–71. With chromosome investigation. *Ann. Hum. Genet.* 40:177, 1976.

# CHAPTER XVIII

# Amniocentesis in late pregnancy

Jan Fog Pedersen and Per Ib Jørgensen

## THE AMNIOTIC FLUID

The amniotic fluid surrounding the fetus is not a stagnant pool. The fetus swallows large amounts (near term 400–500 ml per day), and the same volume is replaced by similar amounts of fetal urine. In addition the fluid is distributed to the fetal lungs, even to the lung alveoli.

For that reason the amniotic fluid is a repository for a number of cellular and biochemical compounds, excreted from the fetal urinary, respiratory and alimentary tracts. Today, many of these important compounds indicating the condition of the fetus have been identified. Consequently several amniotic fluid assays have been established in the daily clinic, and new assays have great possibilities of succeeding.

## METHOD OF EXAMINATION

The clinical value of diagnostic amniocentesis during late pregnancy has to be seriously weighed against risks to the mother and the fetus.

Without ultrasound there is no meaningful way of avoiding penetration of the placenta with the risks of bleeding and feto-maternal transfusion. Therefore ultrasonic scanning should be used for localizing the placenta and for guiding the puncture.

When preparing for amniocentesis, a pocket of amniotic fluid is searched for, which can be reached without hitting the fetus, and ideally without traversing the placenta. We do not at all want to penetrate the placenta in third trimester amniocentesis, and this leaves us with approximately 10% of the cases where amniocentesis is impossible. The typical situation is that of an anterior placenta with the fetal trunk lying below the only placenta-free window. In these cases it may be possible to lift the fetal head out of the pelvis and perform a suprapubic tap, whereas only rarely is it possible to push the fetus and create a pocket

of fluid behind its back. When we feel that the benefits from the procedure outweigh the risks we will deliberately traverse the placenta.

Clearly, the puncture transducer with the central canal could be used to direct the needle to the desired position in the intrauterine cavity. This way of guiding amniocentesis shall not be discussed further in this chapter. Instead two alternative techniques shall be described, one guided by dynamic scanning and the other by conventional B-scanning without the use of a puncture transducer.

## Amniocentesis guided by dynamic scanning

A multielement transducer is mounted in a perspex frame, one end of which fits a perspex puncture adaptor (Fig. 18.1). This contains an adjustable block with a central canal, which will guide the needle in the scanning plane, but in an adjustable angle to the transducer face. Angulations of 30, 45 and 60 degrees are marked on the puncture adaptor, and corresponding oblique lines are drawn on the oscilloscope. The puncture adaptor is sterilized in the same manner as the conventional one.

The uterus is scanned and the optimum site of puncture is chosen and marked on the skin. The correct angle for the guiding canal of the adaptor is read from the oscilloscope and adjusted, and the skin is sterilized. The sterilized puncture adaptor is mounted on the transducer, which is then wrapped in sterile adhesive dressing, leaving the main part of the puncture adaptor free. The sterile transducer-adaptor assembly is placed on the skin, the needle is introduced through the guide canal and inserted at the mark on the skin. The needle should be sharp, optimally a disposable needle and it should be inserted with a rapid movement. The

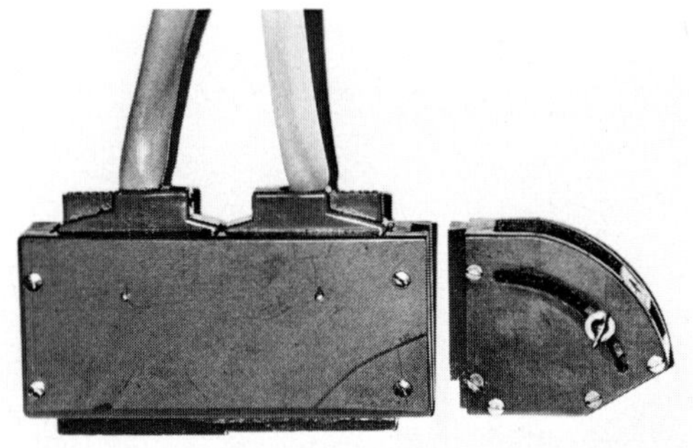

Fig. 18.1. *Multielement transducer and puncture adaptor*
Left, multielement transducer in frame of perspex. Right, puncture adaptor with adjustable block with puncture canal.

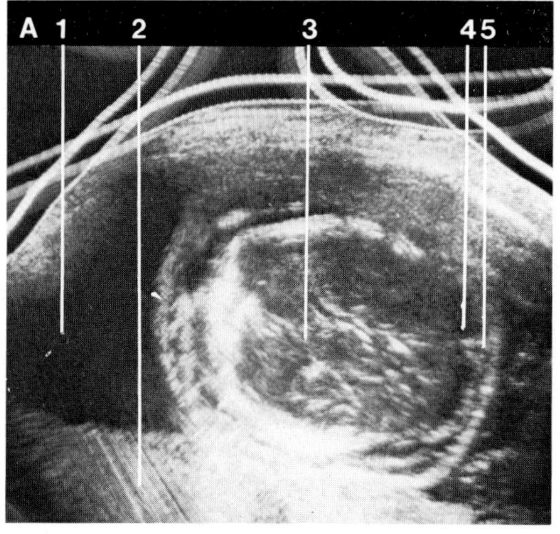


B

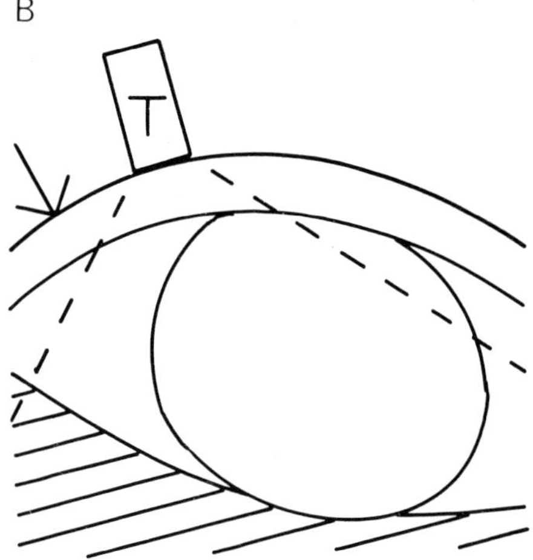


Fig. 18.3. *Amniocentesis guided by conventional B-scanning*
A. Transverse scan. 1. Amniotic fluid, 2. Posterior placenta, 3. Fetal abdomen, 4. Ascites, 5. Thickened edematous abdominal wall. B. Sketch showing puncture site (arrow) and position of transducer (T) allowing scanning of the puncture area.

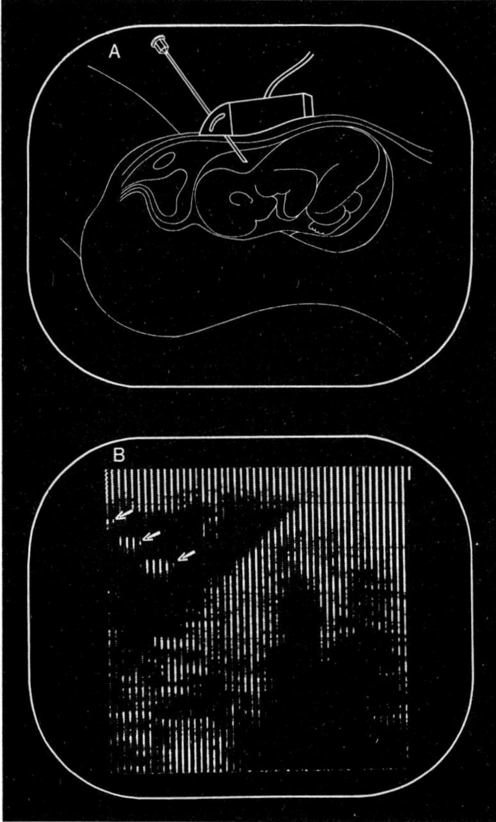


Fig. 18.2. *Amniocentesis guided by dynamic scanning*
A. Sketch showing needle inserted through puncture adaptor into amniotic fluid. B. Dynamic scan showing strong reflections from the needle (arrows).



Amniocentesis in late pregnancy

needle will now follow the corresponding line on the oscilloscope and may thus be advanced to the desired position under direct monitoring, and the aspiration can be performed, also under direct monitoring (Fig. 18.2).

## Amniocentesis guided by conventional B-scanning

This technique requires an ultrasound B-scanner, a skin marker, iodine, a needle and a syringe, but no assistant. Fig. 18.3 A shows a transverse scan of a typical fetus in erythroblastosis, with the edematous, thickened abdominal wall and a little ascites. The optimum site of puncture is chosen and marked on the skin. The transducer is placed on the skin approximately 5 cm away, so that it can be angled to scan the area below the puncture site (Fig. 18.3 B). The skin at the puncture site is rinsed from oil, sterilized, and just before puncture the area below is scanned to ensure that the fetus has not moved in below the puncture site. Then the needle is inserted and the aspiration performed. The small disposable needle, gauge 20, 65 mm long, causes very little pain and also very little irritation to the uterus. No local anesthetic is applied to the skin.

In a series of 174 third trimester amniocenteses mainly requested in patients with diabetes mellitus or Rh disease, amniocentesis without penetrating the placenta was considered impossible in 16 or 11%. Among the remaining 158 cases the success rate was 97%. Clearly, these two figures are interconnected. A higher rate of unworkable punctures will result in a higher success rate of the attempted ones, and vice versa. The question is to find the balance and know when to puncture and when not.

In most of the patients where amniocentesis was considered impossible, there was some small pocket of fluid which probably could have been tapped by using the puncture transducer to guide the needle.

## CLINICAL ASPECTS

Thanks to the ultrasound technique, amniocentesis plays a major and still increasing role as a diagnostic tool in prenatal medicine.

Amniocentesis performed during *early pregnancy* is designed to diagnose developmental disorders of the fetus in time for preventive interruption of pregnancy. For that reason the incidence of severe congenital anomalies among newborns and grown-up children has been reduced considerably (chromosomal disorders, sex-linked diseases, neural tube defects, inborn errors of metabolism). For further details, see chapter XVII.

During *late pregnancy* the main purpose of amniotic fluid assays is to secure a normal fetal development, growth and maturation, in other words:

To prevent perinatal death and to prevent irreversible fetal damage, and consequently mental retardation, spastic paralysis and other neurological defects.

## FETAL HEMOLYTIC DISEASE

In the case of feto-maternal blood group incompatibility, fetal red blood cells are destroyed by an antibody of maternal origin. The two major groups of antigens responsible for fetal hemolytic disease, are the Rh and ABO groups. Of the two, Rh-incompatibility is by far the more severe. It has been responsible for a very high fetal mortality (hydrops fetalis) and a significant neonatal morbidity and mortality (severe anemia, hyperbilirubinemia and neurologic damage secondary to bilirubin encephalopathy (Kernicterus)).

During the 1960s two major advances in fetal medicine occurred in the areas of prevention and treatment of fetal hemolytical disease:

## Amniocentesis

The amniotic fluid concentration of bilirubin is, to a very high degree, correlated to the severity of fetal hemolytic disease. The initial amniocentesis may be performed as early as the 24th week of pregnancy and may be repeated at 1- or 2-week intervals. A high bilirubin level may indicate treatment, consisting of intrauterine transfusion or immediate delivery. It is dependent on the degree of fetal pulmonary maturity assessed by determining the quantity of surface active phospholipids in amniotic fluid (see page 94).

## Intrauterine transfusion

The basic principle of intrauterine transfusion is the treatment of the profound anemia of the fetus with packed red blood cells, injected into the fetal peritoneal cavity, and absorbed into the fetal circulation.

Intrauterine transfusion is performed traditionally after amniography and *radiographic localization*, utilizing fluoroscopy, of the needle and the needle puncture site into the fetal abdominal wall. Complications of this procedure are trauma to the placenta, the umbilical cord and to fetal organs such as the kidney and liver. *Ultrasound guided* intrauterine transfusion, eliminates any factor of placement uncertainty, and the risks of inducing fetal damage are reduced.

# FETAL LUNG IMMATURITY, RESPIRATORY DISTRESS SYNDROME (RDS)

Preterm termination of pregnancy by induction of labor or Caesarean section is an important therapeutic decision in obstetrics. It may be indicated for fetal well-being (Rh-isoimmunization, intrauterine growth retardation) or for both fetal and maternal well-being (toxemia, hypertension, diabetes mellitus). However, selection of the optimal time for preterm termination of pregnancy requires an ability to estimate the degree of fetal maturation.

The major immediate problem facing the premature newborn is respiratory function, and for that reason tests reflecting lung maturity are particularly valuable.

## The respiratory distress syndrome (RDS)

RDS is an acute disorder of the premature infant and by far the most important life-threatening illness among newborns. Clinical signs, which usually appear shortly after birth, include retraction of the chest wall, expiratory grunt and cyanosis. The clinical course usually lasts from 3 to 5 days, ending in recovery of the infant or death. The mortality rate from this disorder has been estimated to be between 30% and 60%! Atelectasis of the alveoli is observed in all infants dying with RDS. These findings have been correlated with the lack of pulmonary surfactant, a surface-active phospholipid that maintains alveolar stability and prevents their collapse at the end of expiration (atelectasis).

Lung secretions contribute to the formation of amniotic fluid, and the phospholipid composition of both fluids is identical. Therefore the concentration of surface-active phospholipids in amniotic fluid correlates to the production of phospholipids by the fetal lung.

## Amniotic fluid surfactant tests

**The Lecithin-Sphingomyelin ratio (L/S ratio)**
Lecithin is the principal pulmonary surfactant, synthesized by the alveolar cells.

Sphingomyelin lacks surfactant properties. The L/S ratio is 1 or less until 30–32 weeks' gestation and reaches 2 at approximately 35 weeks and continues to increase to term.

A L/S ratio of less than 1.0 is always predictive of severe RDS. A ratio of 1.0 to 1.49 is associated with a less severe form of RDS. Ratios of 1.50 to 1.99 may or may not be associated with RDS, whereas ratios of 2.00 or more are almost never associated with the RDS.

**Other surfactant tests**
Other tests for amniotic fluid surfactant include the measurement of lecithin, total phospholipids, palmatic acid and the palmatic acid/stearic acid ratio.

Rapid screening tests include the shake test (bubble stability test) and measurement of the optical density and the fluorescent polarization of the amniotic fluid.

However, the L/S ratio is still the fetal lung maturity test second to none.

## Antenatal prevention of RDS

The first principle in modern obstetrics is to avoid permanent fetal damage. For that reason signs of imminent danger to the fetus (e.g. erytroblastosis and fetal growth retardation) may indicate preterm termination of pregnancy. If the L/S ratio shows that the fetal lungs are mature, the infant is better off outside than inside the uterus. If the L/S ratio is less than 2, RDS is prevented by the administration of corticosteroids to the mother, usually by injection of betamethasonum 12 or 8 mg daily for 3 days.

For that reason the incidence of RDS as well as the perinatal mortality rate and the incidence of permanent fetal damage have been reduced considerably.

## THE FUTURE

*Intrafetal transfusions* and *therapeutic injections* direct to the fetus (see chapter XIX) have already been established. Furthermore there is every chance to believe in *direct nutrition of the fetus* by intraamniotic infusion of essential compounds (e.g. amino acids), swallowed and resorbed by the undernourished, starving fetus (severe placental dysfunction).

# References


Bang, J. and Northeved, A.: A new ultrasonic method for transabdominal amniocentesis. *Am. J. Obstet. Gynecol.* 114:599, 1972.

Behrman, R. E.: Neonatal-Perinatal Medicine. Diseases of the fetus and infant. *C. V. Mosby,* Saint Louis, 1977.

Curtis, J. D., Cohen, W. N., Richerson, H. B. and White, C. A.: The importance of placental localization preceding amniocentesis. *Obstet. Gynecol.* 40:194, 1972.

Evans, H. E. and Glass, L.: Perinatal medicine. *Harper & Row,* Hagerstown, New York, San Francisco, London, 1976.

Frigoletto, F. D., Joson, C. B., Rothchild, S. B., Finberg, H. J. and Umansky, I.: Intrauterine transfusion with the use of phased array ultrasonography: A new technique. *Am. J. Obstet. Gynecol.* 131:273, 1977.

Gluck, L., Kulovich, M. V., Barer, R. C., Brenner, P. H., Andersson, C. C. and Spellacy, V. N.: Diagnosis of the respiratory distress syndrome by amniocentesis. *Am. J. Obstet. Gynecol.* 109:440, 1971.

Goodlin, R. C.: Care of the Fetus. *Masson Publishing Inc.,* New York, 1979.

Liggins, G. C. and Howie, R. N.: A controlled trial of antepartum glucocorticoid treatment for prevention of respiratory distress syndrome in premature infants. *Pediatrics* 50:515, 1972.

Pedersen, J. F.: Percutaneous puncture guided by ultrasonic multitransducer scanning. *J. Clin. Ultrasound* 5:175, 1977.

# CHAPTER XIX

# Intrauterine injections

Jørgen Falck Larsen

The ultrasonically guided puncture technique permits injection into the uterine contents:
1) Injection into the amniotic fluid
2) Injection into the placenta
3) Injection into the fetus.

## INJECTION INTO THE AMNIOTIC FLUID

Prostaglandin $F_{2\alpha}$ is an efficient drug in *termination of pregnancy* in the second trimester. Intraamniotic administration seems to be the most acceptable method. After the 14th week of gestation, prostaglandin can be injected "blindly", but between the 12th and 14th week ultrasonically guided puncture is preferable. We use the technique after the 14th week as well to avoid lesions with the risk of feto-maternal transfusion and possible immunization.

A multitransducer scanner with a central puncture canal is used. The fetus, placenta and needle tip are visible on the scanning picture. A small amount of amniotic fluid is aspirated to make sure that the needle is placed in the amniotic cavity, and 40 mg prostaglandin $F_{2\alpha}$ is then injected into the amniotic fluid.

Another important application is injection of contrast media for *amniography*. After aspiration of amniotic fluid, two contrast media are injected:

(a) Urografin[R] (meglumini amidotrizoas 75%) 15 ml, and Lipoidol[R] (lipoidol ethylique fluid) 6 ml. The water soluble Urografin will be swallowed by the fetus and make the fetal intestines visible (Fig. 19.1) while the oily Lipoidol demonstrates the surface of the fetus due to adhesiveness to the fat of the skin.

This method is used in combination with high resolution dynamic ultrasound scanning when fetal malformations are suspected, such as cases with low plasma estrogen or high alpha-feto-protein.

The fetus swallows the amniotic fluid: It is absorbed by the intestinal villi and enters the fetal

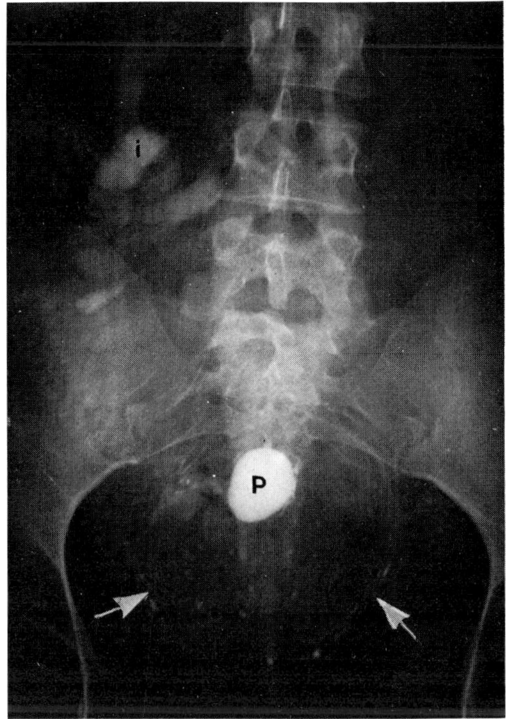


Fig. 19.1. *Normal amniography*
The Urografin injected into the amniotic cavity has been swallowed by the fetus and is seen in the intestines (i). The oily Lipoidol is demonstrating the surface of the fetus (white arrows). Some of the Lipoidol has not been fixed to the skin of the fetus and is concentrated in a pool in the amniotic fluid (P).

circulation. Between the 20th and 30th weeks the fetal skin is poorly developed and a diffusion takes place through the skin. The fetal urine forms the main source of the liquor amnii. This interchange between amniotic fluid and fetal circulation opens an interesting new field of *feeding and medication of the fetus*. Theoretically, it should be possible to supply essential materials to the fetus in cases of placental insufficiency by injecting the materials into the amniotic fluid. It is also possible to carry out metabolic and endocrinological tests by offering a material to the fetus by an intraamniotic injection and measure the metabolites in the amniotic fluid or maternal plasma. These methods, however, are still at an experimental stage.

## INJECTION INTO THE PLACENTA

This application has no clinical value at present. It may be possible to develop a method for *"placental clearance"*, but a technical problem is to place the needle into the maternal blood pool without lesion of the villus with the risk of fetal-maternal transfusion.

## INJECTION INTO THE FETUS

Intramuscular injection into the gluteal region of the fetus is not very difficult. The method has been developed in the ultrasound laboratories of Gentofte and Herlev hospitals.

The gluteal region of the fetus is identified and – under sterile conditions – a guided needle with an outer diameter of 1.2 mm is introduced through the abdominal wall and the uterine wall. When the guide needle is placed in the uterine cavity, a thin needle is inserted through the guide needle and advanced into the fetal gluteal region. When placed into the fetal buttock, the injection is performed (Fig. 19.2).

The newborn infants should be examined for possible injurious effects and the injection marks recorded. We found no injurious effect and the injection marks confirmed that all fetuses had injections in the gluteal region.

The application of this technique could be illustrated by two examples: 1) injection of vitamin-K into fetuses where the mother had received anticoagulant therapy, 2) injection of corticosteroids into the fetus to prevent respiratory distress syndrome (RDS),

### Injection of vitamin-K

Thromboembolic disease is a serious complication to pregnancy. Anticoagulant therapy has reduced the risk of maternal death. On the other hand the use of anticoagulants exposes the mother as well as the fetus to the hazard of hemorrhage. The maternal complications are not severe, but the fetus is exposed to great risk as the anticoagulant passes the placental barrier and may cause hemorrhage in the brain of the infant during delivery.

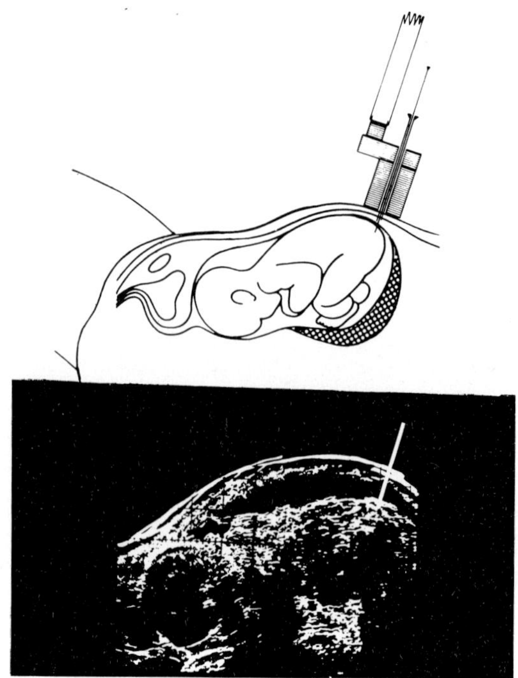

Fig. 19.2. *Ultrasonically guided injection into the gluteal region of the fetus*

As the anti-K-vitamin drugs pass the placental membrane, it has been suggested to use heparin, which – with a molecular weight of 16,000 – does not pass the placental membrane and therefore does not change the coagulation status of the fetus and infant.

The heparin treatment is, however, difficult to control for a long period. Therefore, the anticoagulant therapy may be designed as a combination of the two methods using an oral anticoagulant of the anti-vitamin K-type until 37th week of gestation followed by heparin until after delivery. Theoretically, this allows the fetus to eliminate the anti-K-vitamin before delivery, reducing the risk of hemorrhage.

Spontaneous recovery of a normal coagulation status is very slow. Fig. 19.3 shows that the coagulation status was very poor in cases in which a spontaneous recovery was expected. The situation was not improved by intravenous and intraamniotic injections of vitamin-K 2–4 days prior to delivery. Therefore, it was decided to inject vitamin-K into the gluteal region of the fetus. We used 2.5 to 3.0 mg phytomenandion. It was tried in four cases and in all cases the effect was much better than

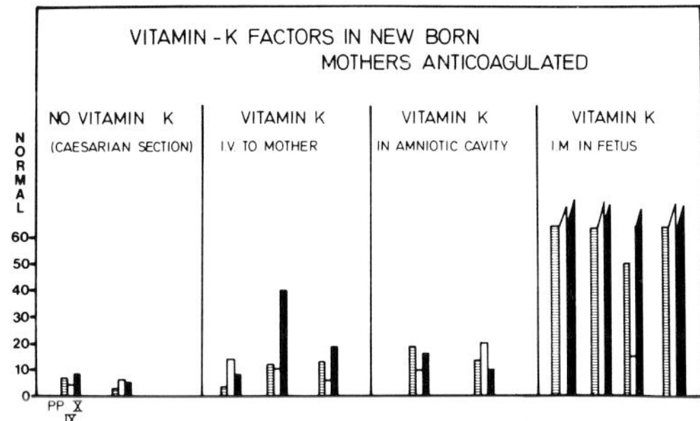


Fig. 19.3. *Coagulation factors of newborns after treatment of the mothers with anti-K-vitamin*
If no K-vitamin was given, the factors were very low. The factors were not improved very much by injection of K-vitamin intravenously to the mother or intraamniotic injection. After injection into the fetus the factors were almost normal.

in cases with intravenous or intraamniotic vitamin-K.

In three of the four cases the interval between the injection and the delivery was more than 36 hours. In these cases the coagulation status was normal. In one case the interval was shorter and the coagulation was improved, but not normal. All infants survived without signs of hemorrhage. Therefore, we recommend the injection to be performed 36 hours before delivery.

## Injection of corticosteroid

Respiratory distress syndrome (RDS) is a serious condition responsible for many deaths in preterm infants. Prevention of this syndrome is especially important in cases of premature rupture of the membranes or in induction of labor in cases with uncertain gestational age.

Determination of the relation between lecitin and sphingomyelin in the amniotic fluid (L/S ratio, see page 94) reflects the maturation of the surfactant of the fetal lungs. An L/S ratio below 2.1, indicates that the fetal lungs are immature and the risk of RDS is considerable.

In animal experiments the maturation of the lung surfactant may be accelerated by corticosteroids. We have confirmed this in the human by injecting 2.5 – 5.0 methyl prednisolon per estimated kg fetal weight into the fetus. In most cases one injection was enough to produce fetal lung maturity evaluated by the L/S ratio, but in two cases the injection had to be repeated.

Later investigations demonstrated that the corticosteroids passed the placental membrane. Therefore, it is much simpler to give the corticosteroid to the mother, and the method has no clinical importance. However, it showed that medication of the fetus is easy using the direct injection technique.

Therefore, this method may be used in all cases in which the fetus needs treatment with a substance which does not pass the placental membrane.

## References


Falck Larsen, J., Jacobsen, B., Holm, H. H., Pedersen, J. F. and Mantoni, M.: Intrauterine injection of vitamin K before the delivery during anticoagulant therapy of the mother. *Acta Obstet. Gynecol. Scand.* 57:227, 1978.

Nielsen, K. R., Gregersen, E., Falck Larsen, J. and Olsen, C. E.: Prostaglandin F₂ and oxytocin compared with hypertonic saline and oxytocin for the induction of second trimester abortion. *Acta Obstet. Gynec. Scand. Suppl.* 37:57, 1975.

Russel, J. G. B.: Amniography and fetography. Radiology in Obstetrics and Antenatal Pediatrics, *Butterworths*, London 1973. p. 10.

Verder, H., Feldbo, M., Fonseca, G., Hancke, S., Jørgensen, P. I., Falck Larsen, J. and Vang, N.: Lecithin-sphingomyelin ratio in amniotic fluid for determination of the optimal time of termination of pregnancy. *Dan. Med. Bull.* 25:212, 1978.

# CHAPTER XX

# Miscellaneous ultrasonically guided punctures

Flemming Jensen

## THYROID PUNCTURE

At ultrasonic scanning, complete two dimensional sectional mapping of the gland is obtained, thereby enabling a morphological diagnosis of a palpable mass: is it a smooth-walled cyst, an inhomogenous solid lesion or a mixed cystic/solid lesion?

Fig. 20.1 shows a relatively large (2 cm) solitary smooth-walled cyst in the left thyroid lobe.

It is easy to determine ultrasonically whether a lesion of this size is cystic or solid. A nodular nontoxic goiter in the left lobe of the thyroid is seen in Fig. 20.2. The interior echo configuration is inhomogenous with a mixture of dense solid areas and small cystic cavities.

The precise outlining and demonstration of the interior of a thyroid lesion with distinction between cystic and solid areas give the examiner the optimal chance of obtaining representative biopsies.

With solid or mixed lesions a certain risk of malignancy exists and it has been shown that clinical signs are practically without value regarding this risk. Moreover, a preoperative biopsy according to different authors shows false negative results in 8–33%. Especially the highly differentiated follicular carcinoma may be impossible to diagnose cytologically and even histologically as it mimics normal thyroid tissue or an adenoma. Even in evaluation of operatively obtained, frozen sections the false negative rate has been shown to be about 12%. These facts indicate that proper treatment of patients with proven solid or mixed lesions is very difficult.

Until now the most valuable use of ultrasonically guided fine-needle puncture in thyroid diagnosis is in the handling of patients with simple cysts, who may be spared an operation. A small cyst may cosmetically and in other respects be

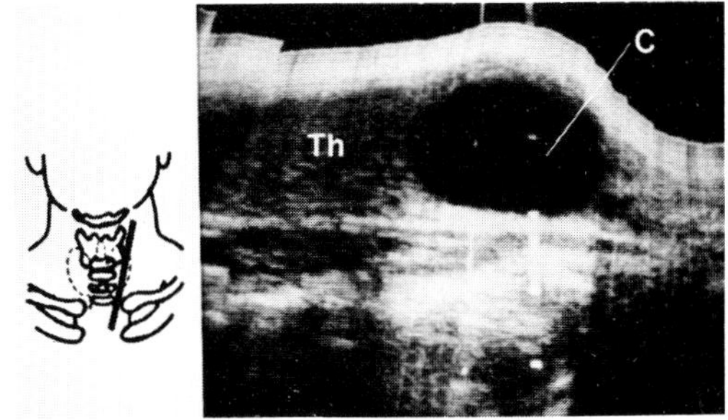

Fig. 20.1. *Ultrasonic scan of thyroid cyst*
Simple solitary cyst in the left thyroid lobe. Th: Thyroid tissue, C: cyst.

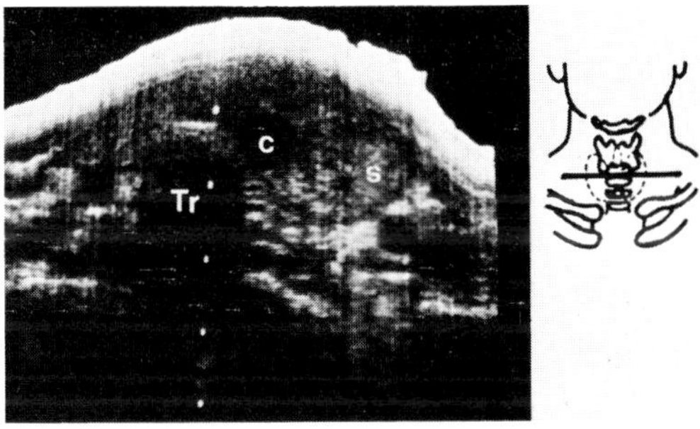

Fig. 20.2. *Ultrasonic scan of complex focal thyroid lesion*
Tr: Trachea, c: cystic component, s: solid component.

acceptable to the patient, provided the benign nature of the lesion can be assured.

In a personal series approximately 25% of the cysts disappeared after the puncture, which means that aspiration may also be of therapeutic value. Figs. 20.3 to 20.6 show some typical cytological aspirates from various types of thyroid focal lesions.

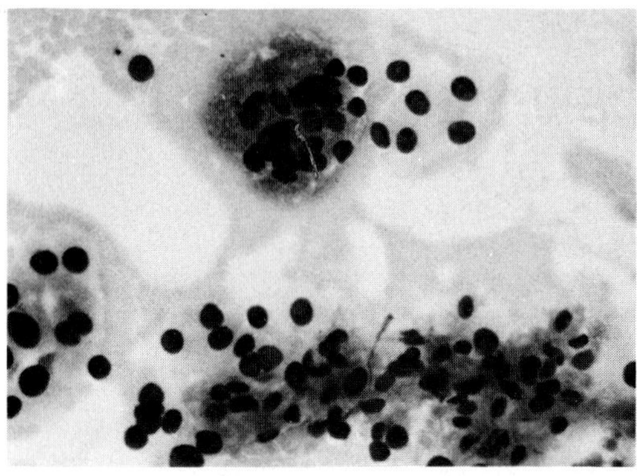

Fig. 20.3. *Fine needle aspirate from thyroid adenoma*
Clusters of rounded cells of almost uniform size. There is no suspicion of malignancy.

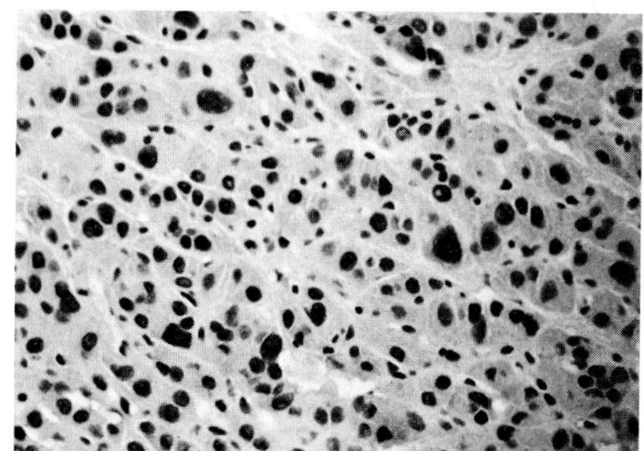

Fig. 20.6. *Thyroid carcinoma histology*
A histological section of the removed thyroid of which the cytological aspirate in Fig. 20.5. originates. It was finally classified as an oncocytoma with focal malignancy.

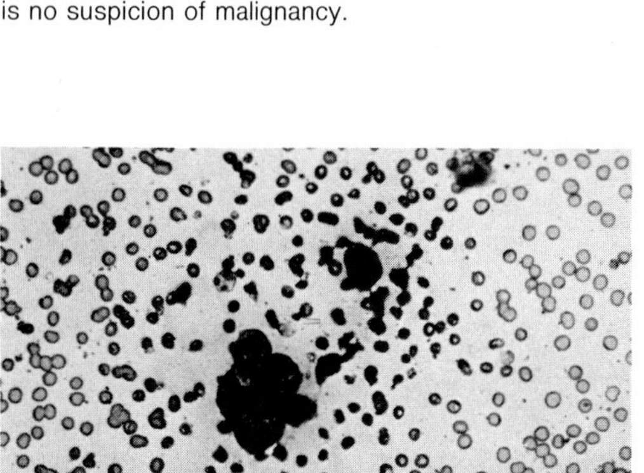

Fig. 20.4. *Aspirate from benign thyroid cyst*
Macrophages containing granula of pigment are seen surrounded by erythrocytes. In some cases also cells from the epithelium of the cyst wall may be demonstrated.

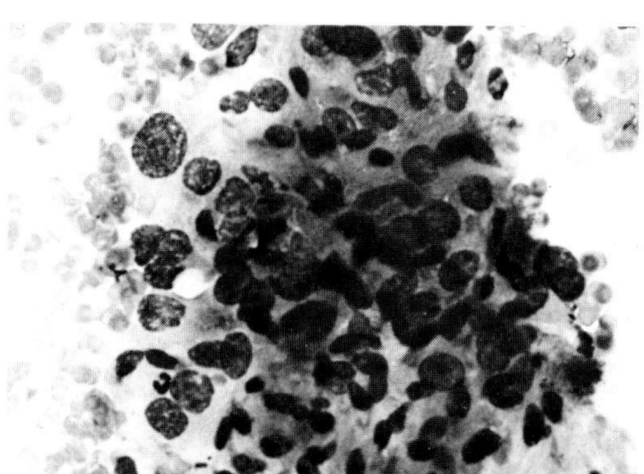

Fig. 20.5. *Fine needle aspirate from thyroid cancer*
Cells of most varying size and shape, some with large nucleoli, are seen.

# PUNCTURE OF THE URINARY BLADDER

Suprapubic puncture of the urinary bladder for diagnostic or therapeutic purposes can be done safely under ultrasonic guidance, when percussion of the bladder damping is equivocal.

A longitudinal scan in the midline will clearly demonstrate the extent of bladder wall in contact with the anterior abdominal wall above the symphysis pubis. (Fig. 20.7). A needle or a catheter can then be introduced. In almost all cases this can be done safely without the use of a special puncture transducer.

# PLEURO- AND PERICARDIOCENTESIS

Ultrasonically guided pleurocentesis or pericardiocentesis minimizes the risk of lung and heart injury. An intercostal route may be chosen according to the scans. Fig. 20.8 shows an echo-poor, circumscribed lesion in contact with the anterior thoracic wall posteriorly surrounded by air-containing lung tissue. Percutaneous puncture proved it to be an abscess.

When dealing with free or loculated pleural fluid, the optimal intercostal space for puncture, can be chosen; that is the most dependent point, where the fluid collection has a reasonable depth. The needle may be introduced without or through a puncture transducer and be retracted slowly until virtually all fluid is aspirated or a soft plastic catheter may be introduced.



Miscellaneous

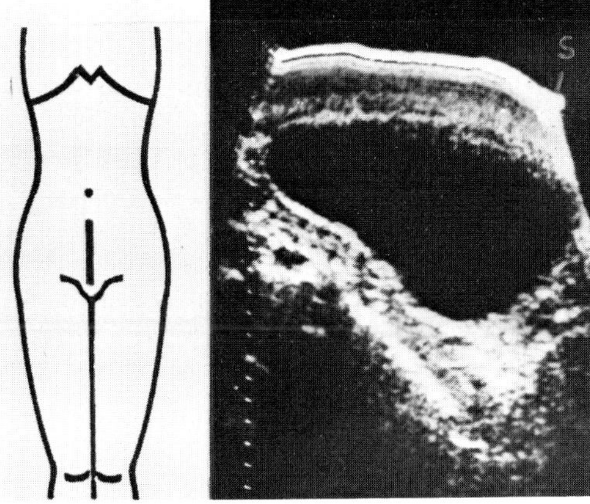

Fig. 20.7. *Ultrasonic scan of the urinary bladder*
Scan through lower abdomen in the mid-sagittal plane. The urinary bladder containing approximately 400 ml, is seen to extend well above the symphysis pubis(s).

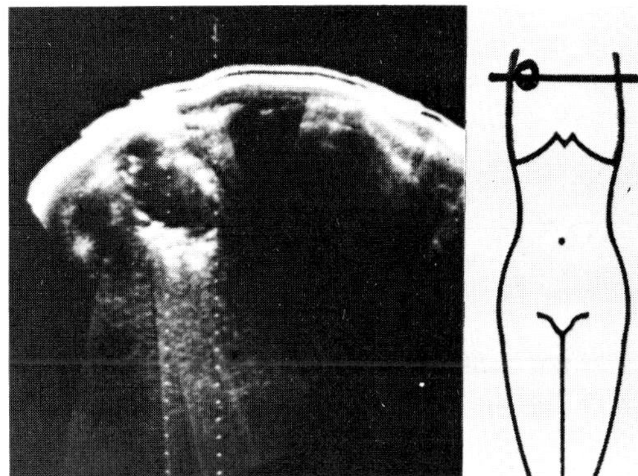

Fig. 20.8. *Ultrasonic scan of lung abscess*
Transverse scan of a pulmonary fluid-filled, circumscribed lesion in contact with the anterior wall of the right hemithorax.

This will further reduce the risk of pneumothorax or myocardial perforation and secure a more complete emptying.

Usually an A-mode image is sufficent to find a proper point to introduce a needle into the pericardial space.

The use of a puncture transducer is advisable. Depending on the position of the diaphragm, and thereby the liver, a subxiphoid route can be chosen. With large, anteriorly situated effusions an intercostal access may be used.

Instead of A- or TM-mode guidance, monitoring of the procedure may be accomplished with a dynamic scanner, which can achieve sufficient skin contact in an intercostal space.

## PUNCTURE OF VESSELS

Localization of major arteries and veins prior to catherization may be accomplished by means of ultrasonic Doppler equipment. As most of the Doppler devices intended for examination of vessels have an optimal depth range from 0.5 to 5 cm, only rather superficially situated vessels may be located. An example of such a vessel which is non-palpable is the subclavian vein.

Petzoldt and co-workers have reported on facilitated tubulation of the subclavian vein in a larger number of patients with the aid of the Doppler technique. They used a sterilized, detachable needleguide and obtained a high success rate with no serious complications following the procedure.

## PUNCTURE OF THE GALL BLADDER

The use of ultrasonically guided gall bladder puncture is still in its infancy, first and foremost due to fear of bile leak into the peritoneal cavity. In the future it may, however, be demonstrated that direct gall bladder puncture may be of value diagnostically (measuring of the constituents of pure bile) as well as therapeutically (in threatening rupture of an inflamed, obstructed gall bladder). Initial experience seems to indicate that the risk of bile leak is diminished when the puncture needle traverses liver parenchyma before it enters the gall bladder lumen.

I am indepted to Dr. Ella Larsen, chief of Dept. of Pathology, Frederiksborg County Hospital, Hillerød, who supplied the photos of the cytological specimens from thyroid lesions.

# References


Bredahl, E. and Simonsen, J: Routine performance of intra-operative frozen section microscopy, with particular reference to diagnostic accuracy. *Acta Path. Microbiol. Scand. Suppl.* 212:104, 1970.

Goldberg, B. B. and Pollack, H. M.: Ultrasonic aspiration biopsy techniques. *J. Clin. Ultrasound* 4:141, 1976.

Hogan, M. T., Watne, A., Mossburg, W. and Castaneda, W.: Direct injection into the gall bladder in dogs, using ultrasonic guidance. *Arch. Surg.* 111:564, 1976.

Jensen, F. and Rasmussen, S. N.: The treatment of thyroid cysts by ultrasonically guided fine needle aspiration. *Acta Chir. Scand.* 142:209, 1976.

Klapdor, R., Scherer, K., Sepehr, H. and Klöppel, G.: The ultrasonically guided puncture of the gall bladder in animals. *Endoscopy* 9:166, 1977.

Petzoldt, R., Lutz, H., Ehler, R., Kresse, H. and Köhl, W.: Puncture of veins and arteries assisted by ultrasound. *Ultrasound Med. Biol.* 2:331, 1976.

Rygård, J. and Rasmusson, B.: Solitary cold thyroid tumours. Benign or malignant? *Ugeskr. Laeg.* 140:2297, 1978.

Walfish, P. G., Hazani, E., Strawbridge, H. T. G., Miskin, M. and Rosen, I. B.: A prospective study of combined ultrasonography and needle aspiration biopsy in the assessment of the hypofunctioning thyroid nodule. *Surgery* 82:474, 1977.

# CHAPTER XXI

# Is there a risk of spreading cancer by percutaneous fine needle aspiration biopsy?

Hans Henrik Holm and Søren Hancke

It has not been too many years since most clinicians strongly condemned the practice of taking surgical biopsies of malignant lesions. Even well-known surgeons referred to biopsy taking as a criminal act, since it was believed that the prognosis was worsened by incision into a tumor. Even though surgical biopsies now are quite well-accepted everywhere, needle biopsies of malignant lesions are in some places still not considered without risk and are looked upon with some suspicion.

When any invasive procedure for the diagnosis of a malignant tumor has to be evaluated with regard to tumor spread and a possibly aggravated prognosis, it should be determined whether the procedure leads to local tumor spread and/or results in transfer of tumor cells into the blood stream or lymph system, possibly resulting in distant metastases.

## Possible distant spread

It is important to remember that the presence of tumor cells in the blood stream of a patient with a malignant tumor certainly does not mean that metastases are present or will occur at all.

Since 1955 with Engell's systematic work on cancer cells in the blood from the vein draining a tumor region, many investigations have been performed in order to elucidate the prognostic significance of tumor cells in the blood stream. In 1959 Engell found that of 117 patients who survived the postoperative period after operation for colorectal cancer, 55 were alive 5–9 years after. In 28 of these, tumor cells were demonstrated in the blood stream during operation. It was concluded that the presence of tumor cells in the blood is of no prognostic importance.

The extensive literature on the significance of circulating tumor cells has later been reviewed by Goldblatt & Nadel and Salsbury. Although there seems to be no unifying concept or understanding of the biological significance of the phenomenon, the opinion has swung from the concept that the presence of circulating tumor cells was virtually a death warrant, to the idea that such circulating cells are possibly harmless.

If an invasive diagnostic procedure like a biopsy was supposed to carry a risk, then it would be reasonable to presume that the more traumatic the biopsy of the tumor, the higher the risk of tumor spread, locally as well as in remote areas.

However, on the basis of animal experiments, it was shown by Wood in 1919 and by Peterson & Nuttall in 1939 that even the relatively traumatic surgical biopsies carried little, if any, risk.

In 1946 also Maun & Dunning demonstrated that a simple biopsy of transplanted adenocarcinoma as well as squamous cell cancer did not affect the average survival period of rats or increase the percentage of metastases to lymph nodes, lung or bone.

Surgical biopsies are more or less indispensable in the operative management of many patients and it is generally accepted that the risk – if any – is far outweighed by the important information gained by the procedure.

Percutaneous needle biopsy has the obvious advantage that a specific diagnosis may be reached without an operation.

In most cases such a biopsy has been performed with a rather coarse needle (more than 1 mm outer diameter), e.g. a Silvermann needle. This has proved to be totally safe in the vast majority of cases.

In 1954, Robbins et al. studied the clinical course of 1576 patients with breast cancer of whom 543 had aspiration biopsies performed.

They concluded that aspiration biopsy seems to have no effect on long-term survival rates among breast cancer patients.

In 1962, Berg & Robbins reexamined the series above using careful case matching; 370 patients who had aspiration biopsy performed were compared with 370 paired controls. There was no difference in survival rates in the two groups.

In 1967 von Schreeb et al. analyzed the 5-year survival rate in two comparable groups with renal adenocarcinoma: 77 patients were operated upon following puncture (0.75–1.5 mm outer diameter needles) and injection of contrast material into the tumor. This group was matched with 73 controls in whom puncture was not performed. The 5-year survival rate in the punctured group was 70%, in contrast to 38% in the nonpunctured group. This somewhat surprising result at least seems to indicate that puncture of malignant renal tumors does not aggravate the prognosis.

## Possible local spread

Besides the risk of spreading tumor cells into the blood and lymph system in the case of needle biopsy, a risk of seeding tumor cells along the needle tract into the adjacent tissue exists. Even though thousands of coarse needle biopsies have been carried out over the years – in particular with prostatic cancer – such a complication has been described only in very few cases (Clarke et al., Goldman & Samellas, Gibbons et al.).

In order to further minimize the risk of spreading tumor cells, the fine needle aspiration biopsy technique using 0.6 mm needles was developed in Sweden. This technique has been used extensively at many centers by applying various forms of needle guidance (Fig. 21.1).

In 1971 Engzell et al. published their results on needle biopsies (18-gauge needle) of carcinomatous lymph nodes transplanted to 21 rabbits. Simultaneously they examined lymph and blood from the punctured nodes as well as the fluid escaping through the puncture holes into the adjacent tissue. They found no evidence that the biopsy released carcinomatous cells into the lymphatic or blood circulation. However, they found that a relatively small number of cells escaped through the capsular perforations in many cases. This finding contrasts the lack of evidence of local tumor extension in many clinical investigations. It

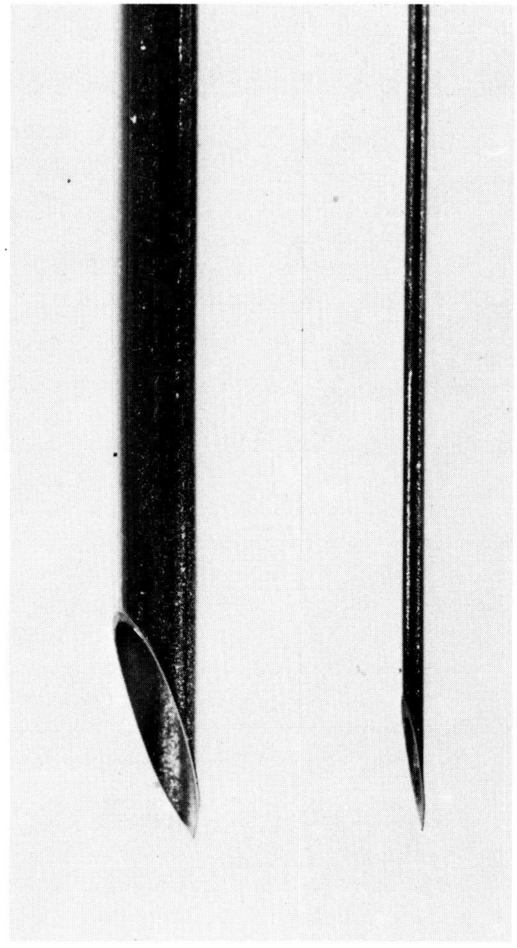

Fig. 21.1. *The tip of a Silverman needle compared to that of a fine needle (23 gauge)*

is therefore likely that tumor cells in the needle tract in almost all cases are destroyed before they can give rise to local tumor growth. In the same publication, clinical follow-up was made of 157 patients with pleomorphic adenomas of the major salivary gland and of 469 patients with prostatic carcinomas, all diagnosed by fine-needle biopsy. In these series no evidence of locally extended growth attributable to the biopsy.

In a series of 4,000 transthoracic fine-needle biopsies in 2,500 patients, Nordenström & Björk found only one documented case and one probable case of metastases implanted in the chest wall.

In a series of 180 malignant tumors of the lung being punctured percutaneously with a fine needle, Francis & Fenger did not find tumor growth attributable to the biopsy.

In 860 patients Lindberg & Åkerman could not demonstrate recurrent tumor growth thought to be the result of the fine-needle aspiration biopsy used.

Franzén (1978), who has used fine-needle aspiration biopsies since the beginning of the 1950s, has experienced only one case of tumor seeding, from a melanoma located centrally in the lung. A few weeks after the puncture, a metastasis developed in the chest wall at the puncture site (same case as mentioned by Nordenström & Björk).

Recently, the second case of tumor seeding using a fine needle has been described. A repeated CT-guided biopsy of a pancreatic cancer using a 22-gauge needle resulted in a subcutaneous metastasis at the puncture site.

At the ultrasonic laboratory at Herlev Hospital (previously Gentofte), almost 1000 ultrasonically guided fine-needle aspiration biopsies of malignant abdominal lesions have been performed since 1969. The tumors were located mainly in the kidneys, pancreas, liver, retroperitoneum and gastrointestinal tract. A 23-gauge needle has been used exclusively for the aspiration biopsies.

Although it is likely that in some cases a small number of malignant cells were spread to the needle tract, we have never experienced locally extended tumor growth which seems to correlate in any way to the fine-needle puncture performed. Whether malignant cells from the tumors were spread to the blood and lymph circulation during the puncture is unknown, but on the basis of the literature, this possibility appears to be of no importance.

It seems justifiable to conclude that the risk of spreading cancer by percutaneous fine-needle aspiration biopsy is more of theoretical than practical significance.

# References


Berg, J. W. and Robbins, G. F.: A late look at the safety of aspiration biopsy. *Cancer* 15:826, 1962.

Burkholder, G. V. and Kaufman, J. J.: Local implantation of carcinoma of the prostate with percutaneous needle biopsy. *J. Urol.* 95:801, 1966.

Clarke, B. G., Leadbetter, W. F. and Campbell, J. S.: Implantation of cancer of the prostate in site of perineal needle biopsy: report of a case. *J. Urol.* 70:937, 1953.

Engell, H. C.: Cancer cells in the circulating blood. *Acta Chir. Scand. Suppl.* 201, 1955.

Engell, H. C.: Cancer cells in the blood: a 5-year follow-up study. *Ann. Surg.* 149:457, 1959.

Engzell, V., Esposti, P. L., Rubio, C., Sigurdson, Å. and Zajicek, J.: Investigation on tumour spread in connection with aspiration biopsy. *Acta Radiologica* 10:385, 1971.

Francis, D. and Fenger, C.: Transtorakal finnålsbiopsi. *Ugeskr. Læger* 138:76, 1976.

Franzén, S., Giertz, G. and Zajicek, J.: Cytological diagnosis of prostatic tumours by transrectal aspiration biopsy: a preliminary report. *Br. J. Urol.* 32:193, 1960.

Franzén, S.: Personal communication, 1978.

Gibbons, R. P., Bush jr., W. H. and Burnett, L. L.: Needle tract seeding following aspiration of renal cell carcinoma. *J. Urol.* 118:865, 1977.

Goldblatt, S. A. and Nadel, E. M.: Cancer cells in the circulating blood: A critical review II. *Acta Cytol.* 9:6, 1965.

Goldman, E. J. and Samellas, W.: Local extension of carcinoma of the prostate following needle biopsy. *J. Urol.* 84:575, 1960.

Lindberg, L. G. and Åkermann, M.: Aspiration cytology of salivary gland tumors: Diagnostic experience from 6-years of routine laboratory work. *Laryngoscope* 86:584, 1976.

Maun, M. E. and Dunning, W. F.: Is the biopsy of neoplasms dangerous? An experimental study. *Surg. Gynecol. Obstet.* 82:567, 1946.

Nordenström, B. and Björk, V. O.: Dissemination of cancer cells by needle biopsy of lung. *Thor. Cardiovasc. Surg.* 65:671, 1973.

Peterson, R. and Nuttall, J. A.: *Am. J. Cancer* 37:64, 1939.

Robbins, G. F., Brothers III, J. H., Eberhart, W. F. and Quan, S.: Is aspiration biopsy of breast cancer dangerous to the patient? *Cancer* 7:774, 1954.

Salsbury, A. J.: The significance of the circulating cancer cells. *Cancer Treatm. Review* 2:55, 1975.

von Schreeb, T., Arner, O., Skovsted, G. and Wikstad, N.: Renal adenocarcinoma. Is there a risk of spreading tumour cells in diagnostic puncture? *Scand. J. Urol. Nephrol.* 1:270, 1967.

Söderström, N.: Fine-needle aspiration biopsy. *Almqvist & Wiksell,* Stockholm, 1966.

Wood, F. C.: *J. Am. Med. Assoc.* 73:764, 1919.

# CHAPTER XXII

# Radio- and chemotherapy follow-up using fine needle biopsies

Hans van der Maase

Abdominal ultrasound is a well-established diagnostic procedure in oncology. The technique is particularly useful in the evaluation of patients with malignant lymfomas and in the assessment and treatment of abdominal metastases from testicular cancer.

Besides the diagnostic application, abdominal ultrasound is used in radiotherapy planning. The technique was first described in 1970, and has shown to be a practical method in the planning of radiation ports and in monitoring progression or regression during radiotherapy.

The tumor response obtained during anticancer chemotherapy can be assessed as well.

Ultrasonically guided fine needle punctures have been performed during the last 10 years and the technique has proved both safe and accurate.

In oncology the fine needle puncture is used in the primary diagnostic evaluation. However, this chapter especially deals with a potential clinical use of fine needle biopsies as a control measure before, during and after radio- and chemotherapy.

Table 22.1. *Tumor size and cytological evaluation before and after radiotherapy*

| Case no. | Diagnosis | Abdominal ultrasound and fine needle biopsy | | | Remarks |
| --- | --- | --- | --- | --- | --- |
| | | Before treatment | 1–2 weeks after radiotherapy | 1–2 months after radiotherapy | |
| I | Testicular seminoma | 8 × 6 × 6 cm + malign. cells | 3 × 4 × 4½ cm no malign. cells | 3 × 4 × 4 cm acellular material | Subsequent operation showed a fibrotic tumor without malignant cells |
| II | | 17 × 9 × 19 cm + malign. cells | no tumor | no tumor | No tumor on subsequent scans |
| III | Testicular teratoma | 3 × 3 × 2 cm + malign. cells | 3 × 2 × 1 cm + malign. cells | no tumor | No tumor on subsequent scans |
| IV | | 6 × 3 × 2 cm + malign. cells | 4 × 1 × 1 cm refused biopsy | no tumor | No tumor on subsequent scans |
| V | | 15 × 5 × 4 cm + malign. cells | 15 × 5 × 3½ cm no malign. cells | 7 × 2½ × 2½ cm no malign. cells | Subsequent scans showed progression and intensive chemotherapy was instituted |
| VI | Colerectal adenocarcinoma | 6 × 4 × 6 cm + malign. cells | 6 × 4 × 6 cm + malign. cells | 4 × 4 × 4 cm no malign. cells | Subsequent laparotomy showed an inoperable malignant tumor |
| VII | | 9 × 12 × 7 cm + malign. cells. | 9 × 11 × 7 cm + malign. cells | 9 × 10 × 7 cm refused biopsy | Subsequent laparotomy showed an inoperable malignant tumor. |
| VIII | | 2 × 2 × 4 cm + malign. cells | 1 × 1 × 3 cm + malign. cells | 1 × 1 × 5 cm acellular material | Subsequent operation showed a fibrotic tumor centrally with few malignant cells. |
| IX | | 7½ × 7 × 5½ cm + malign. cells | 7 × 7 × 5 cm refused biopsy | 3 × 3 × 2 cm refused biopsy | Subsequent scans showed no tumor, confirmed at second-look operation |

# MATERIAL AND METHOD

Nine patients suffering from abdominal tumors have been followed with ultrasonically guided fine needle biopsies before and after radiotherapy or combined radio- and chemotherapy (Table 22.1).

Five patients had testicular cancer with retroperitoneal metastases. In two cases the histological type was a seminoma requiring radiotherapy, and in three cases a teratoma requiring radiotherapy combined with bleomycin and vincristin. Four patients had inoperable colorectal adenocarcinomas. The treatment given was radiation and a combination of 5-fluorouracil, methotrexate and cyclophosphamide. The plan was to perform ultrasonic scanning with fine needle biopsy before, 1–2 weeks and 1–2 months after radiotherapy.

# RESULTS

Before treatment the cytological analysis of the fine needle punctures showed malignant cells in all nine cases (Fig. 22.1).

At first follow-up 1–2 weeks after radiotherapy, there were still malignant cells in four cases and no malignant cells in two cases. It was impossible to have a follow-up of the three remaining patients with fine needle biopsies as two refused, and one was in complete remission at the end of radiotherapy (Fig. 22.2).

At the second follow-up 1–2 months after radiotherapy, there was no tumor left in three cases while two patients refused to have the biopsy performed. The remaining four patients had a fine needle biopsy done. In two of these patients there

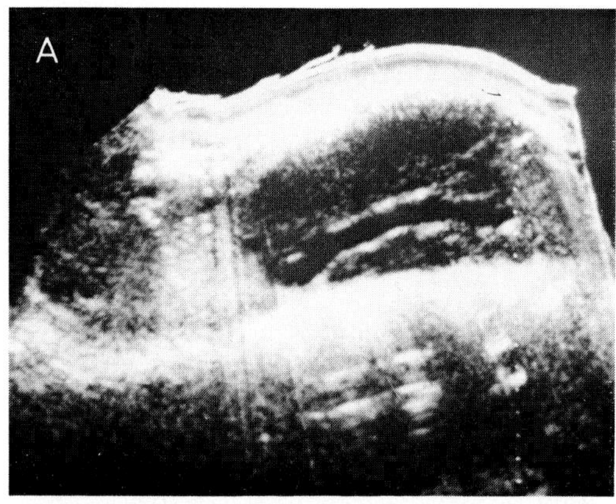

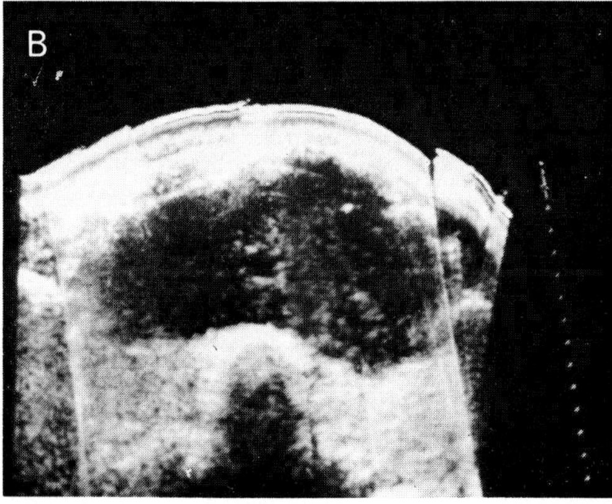

Fig. 22.1. *Testicular seminoma before treatment*
Case no. II from Table 22.I. A. Longitudinal midline scan. B. Transverse scan through midabdomen of a patient with large retroperitoneal lymph node metastases from a testicular seminoma. The aorta is surrounded and displaced by a large mass which measures 17 by 9 by 19 cm. C. Aspirated malignant cells.

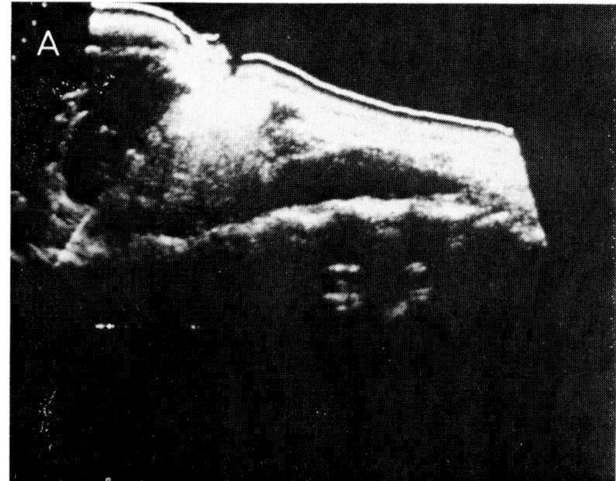

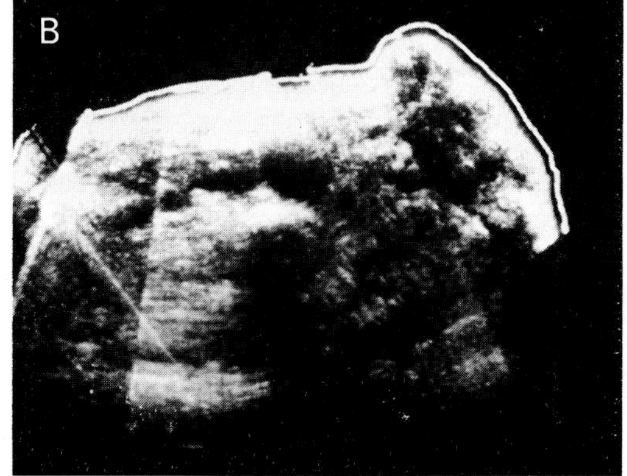

Fig. 22.2. *Testicular seminoma after treatment.*
Case no. II from Table 22.1, 1 week after completed radiotherapy. A. Longitudinal midline scan. B. Transverse midabdominal scan showing complete remission of the tumor (compare with Fig. 22.1).



Radio- and chemotherapy follow-up

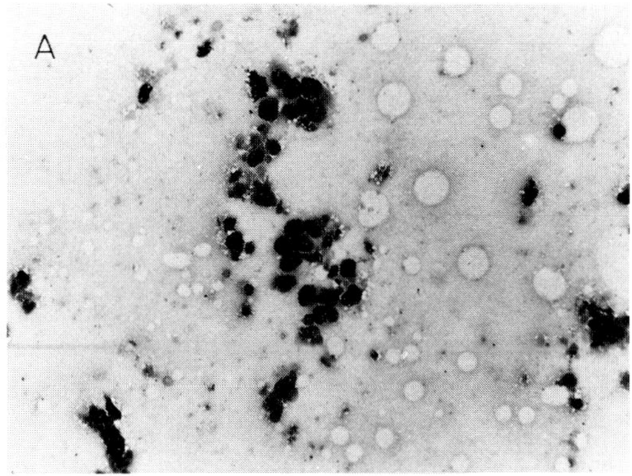

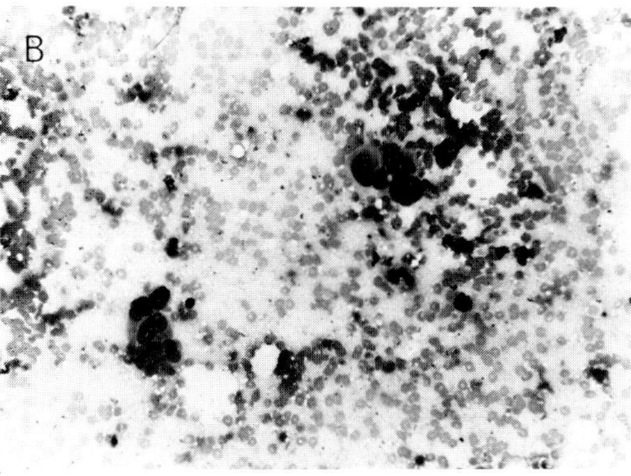

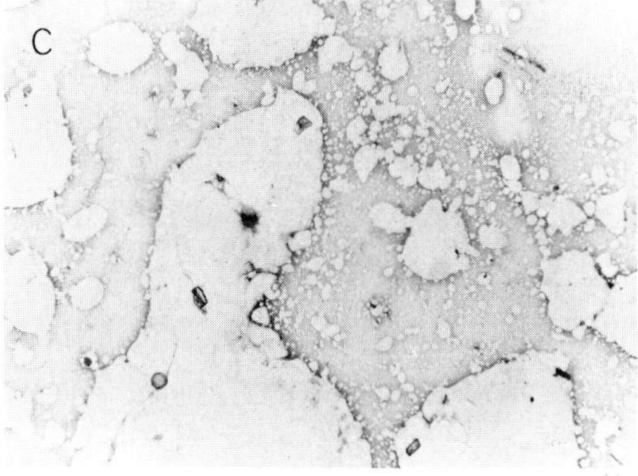

Fig. 22.3. *Aspirated material from colonic adenocarcinoma before and after radiation therapy.*
Case VIII. A. Before treatment obvious malignant cells are found in the aspirate. B. One week after completion of radiation therapy, malignant cells are still found, however, damaged by the irradiation. C. One month later only acellular material is aspirated.

were no malignant cells and in the other two only acellular material was found (Fig. 22.3).

In the two patients with no malignant cells in the the aspirate a later follow-up scan showed progression of the tumor in one and in the other an inoperable malignant tumor was found at subsequent laparotomy. In the two patients with an acellular aspirate the subsequent operation showed a fibrotic tumor without malignant cells in one patient, and a fibrotic tumor with only few malignant cells in the other patient.

## DISCUSSION AND CONCLUSIONS

By controling the effect of radiation or chemotherapy an evaluation of the macroscopic changes of the tumor is generally used.

A more accurate measure would possibly be obtained by evaluating the microscopic changes in the cells during and after treatment, but up til now, there have been no cytological methods which can be used as a routine. The majority of the investigations have been made by evaluation during radiotherapy of benign as well as malignant cells in the vaginal smears from patients with cancer colli uteri.

Some authors have found that the radiation response in these cells has a prognostic significance, but in general the method cannot be used to evaluate the prognosis or as a help in planning the treatment.

The ultrasonically guided fine needle puncture is often used in the diagnostic evaluation of abdominal tumors, but there has been made no systematic investigation of its value as a routine control measure in radio- or chemotherapy.

Considering the small number of patients in this material, the conclusions are therefore partly based on theoretical considerations.

Generally, the ultrasonically guided fine needle puncture is known to be without any inconvenience to the patient. In this material three out of nine patients refused to have the biopsy repeated because of inconvenience at the first or second biopsy. This may very well be due to the fact that this is a very stressed group of patients, considering the malignant diagnosis, treatment, etc. Also it may make a difference if the biopsy is frequently repeated. However it should be no problem, if the biopsy is of value in planning the further treatment.

Before starting treatment, a puncture can ensure that the ultrasonically diagnosed tumor is malignant. However, in most cases this is known beforehand, but if there is doubt, a laparotomy can be avoided by performing a fine needle biopsy.

The main problem is, what decisions concerning further treatment can be made on the basis of a cytologic analysis of material obtained by fine needle biopsies during treatment. Presently progression or regression of tumor size is the decisive factor in the determination of further treatment, and fine needle biopsies are not, at the moment, indicated as a routine during or after radio- and chemotherapy. It must be stressed that this conclusion affects only the routine use of such punctures. There are of course situations where a fine needle biopsy would be of specific interest, but the procedure should be restricted to these situations.

# References


Andersen, J. la Cour: Radiation response i vaginalsekretet. Thesis, Copenhagen 1969.

Asher, W. M. and Freimanis, A. K.: Echographic diagnosis of retroperitoneal lymph node enlargement. *Am. J. Roentgenol.* 105:438, 1969

Brascho, D. J.: Diagnostic ultrasound in radiation treatment planning. *J. Clin. Ultrasound* 1:320, 1973.

Brascho, D. J.: Computerized radiation treatment planning with ultrasound. *Am. J. Roentgenol.* 120:213, 1974

Brascho, D. J., Durant, J. R. and Green, L. E.: The accuracy of retroperitoneal ultrasonography in Hodgkin's disease and non-Hodgkin's lymphoma. *Radiol.* 125:485, 1977.

Filly, R. A., Marglin, S. and Castellino, R. A.: The ultrasonographic spectrum of abdominal and pelvic Hodgkin's disease and non-Hodgkin's lymphoma. *Cancer* 38:2143, 1976.

Graham, R. M. and Graham, J. B.: Cytological prognosis in cancer of the uterine cervix treated radiologically. Cancer 8:59, 1955.

Holm, H. H., Rasmussen, S. N. and Kristensen, J. K.: Ultrasonically guided percutaneous puncture technique. *J. Clin. Ultrasound* 1:27, 1973.

Holm, H. H., Pedersen, J. F., Kristensen, J. K., Rasmussen, S. N., Hancke, S. and Jensen, F.: Ultrasonically guided percutaneous puncture. *Radiol. Clin. North Am.* 13:493, 1975.

Kjellgren, O.: The radiation reaction in the vaginal smear and its prognostic significance. *Acta Radiol.* Suppl. 168. 1958.

Kobayashi, T., Osamutakatani, K., Hattori, N. and Kimura, K.: Echographic evaluation of abdominal tumor regression during antineoplastic treatment. *J. Clin. Ultrasound* 2:131, 1974.

Kobayashi, T., Takatani, O. and Kimura, K.: Echographic patterns of malignant lymphoma. *J. Clin. Ultrasound* 4:181, 1976.

Rochester, D., Bowie, J. D., Kunzmann, A. and Lester, E.: Ultrasound in the staging of lymphoma. *Radiol.* 124:483, 1977.

Rubio, C. A., Hertzberg, O., Kottmeier, H. L., Olsson, E. and Zajicek, J.: Sensitization and radiation response in cases with carcinoma of the uterine cervix. *Acta Radiol.* 3:241, 1965.

Smith, E. H. and Holm, H. H.: Ultrasonic scanning in radiotherapy treatment planning. *Radiol.* 96:433, 1970.

Tyrrel, C. J., Cosgrove, D. O., McCready, V. R. and Peckham, M. J.: The role of ultrasound in the assessment and treatment of abdominal metastases from testicular tumours. *Clin. Radiol.* 28:475, 1977.

# CHAPTER XXIII
# Cytochemistry

## Svend Larsen and Mogens Vilien

In recent years an increasing number of histo- and cytochemical procedures for the identification of intracytoplasmatic cellular components in different cell populations have been developed. The methods, in general, are not established as a routine in pathology, but are for example widely used in hematology parallel to light microscopy examination. By ultrasonically guided puncture technique, it is possible to obtain cellular material from various places in the body. Identification of aspirated cells in such material is sometimes difficult, or in some instances impossible, because the architecture of the tissue is mostly lost. Therefore cytochemical methods applied to the cellular material may supplement light microscopy in differentiating the individual cells. The methods used are directed against cellular products or various intracellular enzyme systems (Table 23.1). Unfortunately, no universal fixative exists to preserve all the different cellular components, and the enzyme activity in particular is very sensitive, not only to the nature of the fixative used, but also to the time of fixation and the temperature (Table 23.2).

The choice of fixative varies according to the cytochemical procedure, but the most commonly used is Baker's formaldehyde calcium chloride (Table 23.3).

Table 23.2. *Changes in enzyme activity related to time and temperature in tissue fixated with 4% formaldehyde-calcium chloride*

| Enzyme | Fixation time (hours) | Temp. (°C) | Activity remaining(%) |
|---|---|---|---|
| Alkaline | 2 | 4 | 73 |
| Phosphatases | 2 | 25 | 35 |
| | 24 | 4 | 26 |
| Acid | 2 | 4 | 79 |
| Phosphatases | 2 | 25 | 40 |
| | 24 | 4 | 50 |
| | 2 | 4 | 82 |
| Esterases | 2 | 25 | 53 |
| | 24 | 4 | 35 |

Table 23.3. *Baker's formaldehyde-calcium chloride*

| | |
|---|---|
| 40% formaldehyde | 150 ml |
| 1.3 g calcium chloride (water free) | 850 ml |
| Time of fixation/temp. | 10 sec–5 min/0–4°C. |

Table 23.1. *Cytoplasmatic contents*

| | | |
|---|---|---|
| Cellular products | Polypeptides | |
| | Carbohydrates | |
| | Mucosubstances | |
| | Amines | |
| | Proteins | |
| | Pigments | |
| | Dehydrogenases | Acid Phosphatases |
| | | Alkaline Phosphatases |
| | | Non-specific Esterases |
| Enzymes | Peroxydases | |
| | Oxydases | |

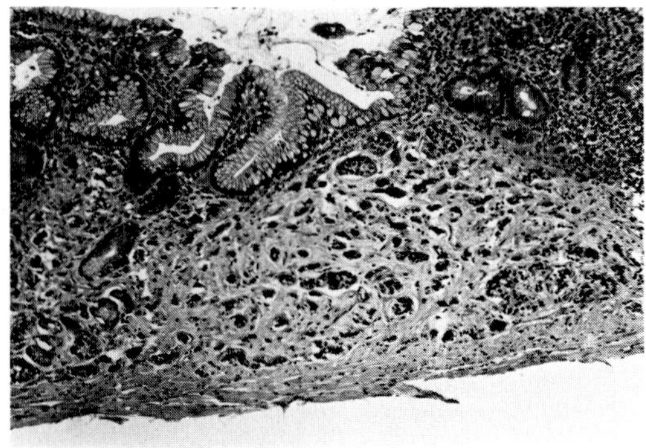

Fig. 23.1. *Zollinger-Ellison syndrome*
The tumor is localized in the gastric mucosa (x 100).

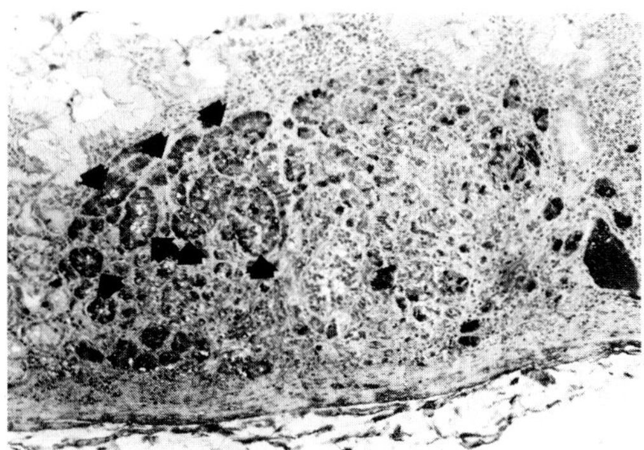

Fig. 23.2. *Zollinger-Ellison syndrome*
Peroxydase conjugated anti-gastrin brownish granula (arrows) bound to the gastrin in the tumor cells.

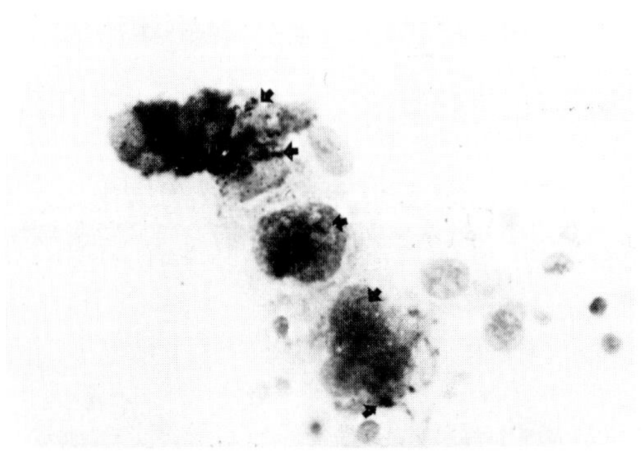

Fig. 23.3. *Osteogenic sarcoma*
Alkaline phosphatases seen as brownish granula in the cytoplasm (arrows). By courtesy of Professor O. Myhre Jensen, Institute of Pathology, Århus Amtssygehus.

Immunochemical procedures with antisera, labeled with fluorescein or conjugated with enzymes, for example horseraddish peroxidase, can be used to identify cells in a specific way by their content of cellular products. Such methods can be applied to formaldehyde-fixated (and paraffin-embedded) material. An increasing number of specific antisera against different cellular products have been developed recently, and can be obtained commercially. Thus, by the use of peroxidase conjugated anti-gastrin, it is possible to identify the gastrin producing cells, for example as shown in a case of Zollinger-Ellison syndrome (Figs. 23.1 and 23.2). The tumor is localized to the gastric mucosa.

In Fig. 23.2 arrows indicate brownish granules produced by peroxidase conjugated anti-gastrin, bound to the gastrin within the cytoplasm of the tumor cells.

In some instances the demonstration of characteristic enzymes in the cells may lead to the diagnosis. In Fig. 23.3 alkaline phosphatases are seen as brownish granules in the cellular cytoplasm. These cells were obtained from a tumor localized in the soft tissue of the lower limb. The diagnosis was an extra-osseous osteogenic sarcoma. The diagnosis could be based solely on the demonstration of alkaline phosphatases in the cells, which were localized in areas where cells containing this enzyme are not normally found.

The distinction between malignant and benign cells in a cellular material by conventional light microscopy is sometimes difficult. Identification of malignant cells based on the demonstration of increased activity of non-specific esterases has been claimed by Bakalos et al. to be of diagnostic value in pleural effusions. A recent blind study by Clausen et al. of 143 serous effusions were investigated for the presence of tumor cells. The material was investigated by conventional cytomorphological methods, and at the same time by staining for non-specific esterases (Figs 23.4 and 23.5). No difference in diagnostic sensitivity was found when the two methods were compared. The low diagnostic sensitivity was caused by intense staining of macrophages and mesothelial cells found in reactive states in the mesothelium.

Cytochemical methods can also be applied to cells kept in tissue culture. An example is shown in Fig. 23.6, where a mixed cell population from ascitic fluid (ovarian carcinoma) bas been cultured

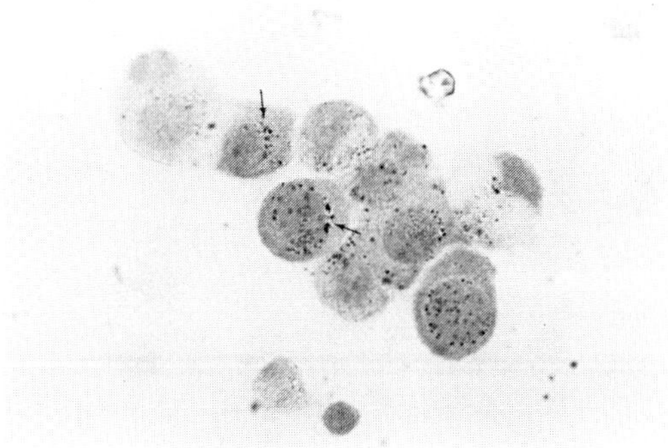

Fig. 23.4. *Slight activity of non-specific esterases in mesothelial cells (arrows)*
By courtesy of Dr. P. P. Clausen, Department of Pathology, Hvidovre Hospital, University of Copenhagen.

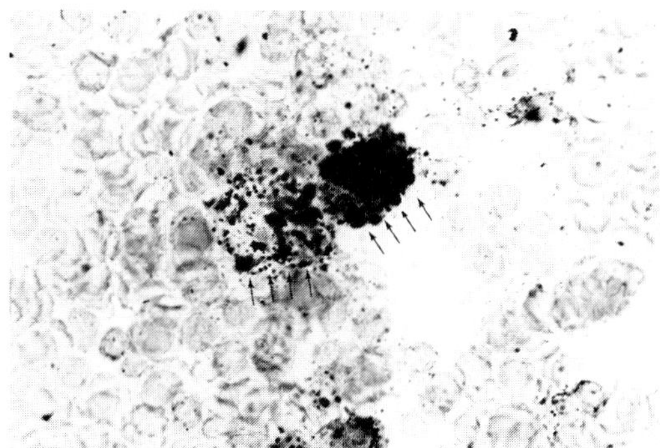

Fig. 23.5. *High activity of non-specific esterases in mesothelial cells (arrows)*
By courtesy of Dr. P. P. Clausen, Department of Pathology, Hvidovre Hospital, University of Copenhagen.

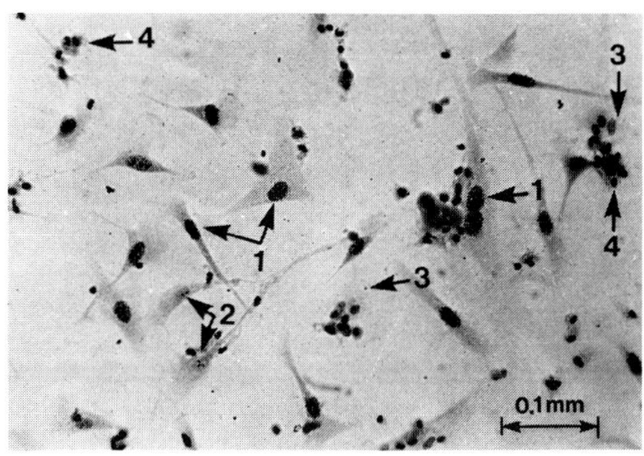


Fig. 23.6. *Tissue culture with [3]H-thymidin incorporation*
1. Large polygonal or elongated cells, possibly tumor cells, with [3]H-labeled nuclei, or 2. Non-labeled nuclei. Together supposedly representing cyclin and non-cycling tumor cells. 3. Non-labeled, medium-sized cells with a rounded cytoplasmic border, possibly macrophages. 4. Small cells with strongly black Giemsa-stained nuclei, must represent adherent leucocytes. Some of the cells may represent other populations, for example, fibroblasts, mesothelium cells or endothelium cells.

on a plastic surface in a tissue culture medium. After 48 hours of cultivation, these cells were labeled with [3]H-thymidine during a further period of 30 hours of cultivation. The cell culture was then fixed, covered with a film, developed and finally fixed and stained with Giemsa. In cells which had been in the S-phase during [3]H-thymidine treatment, the nucleus was covered with fine black spots.

# References


Bakalos, D., Constantakis, N. and Tsicricas, Th.: Recognition of malignant cells in pleural and peritoneal effusions. *Acta. Cytol.* 18:118, 1974.

Clausen, P. P., Højgaard, K. and Tommesen, N.: The diagnostic value of cytochemical staining for non-specific esterase in the search for tumor cells in effusions. *Acta Path. Microbiol. Scand.* A, 87:347, 1979.

Taylor, C. R. and Burns, J.: The demonstration of plasma cells and other immunoglobulin-containing cells in formalin-fixed, paraffin-embedded tissues using peroxidase-labeled antibody. *J. Clin. Path.* 27:14, 1974.

Undritz, E.: Atlas of Haematology, 2nd.ed. *Sandoz*, Basle, 1973.

# CHAPTER XXIV

# Cytoimmunology

## M. Vilien and S. Larsen

Cell material from the human body may be used to monitor the immune state in the organism. The cells can be used for various immune techniques, either as a source of antigen only, as for example in the complement binding reaction and in the lymphocyte transformation test, or as antigen and target cells simultaneously for the immune reaction, as for example in immunofluorescence and cytotoxicity reactions. The cell material, which is obtained by an ultrasonically guided fine needle aspiration biopsy, can be either a small amount of cells from the puncture of a solid mass lesion or a greater number of cells from the puncture of a cyst with cell-containing fluid, or a cellular effusion in a serous cavity, for example the peritoneum.

The cells can be used in various immune techniques to investigate whether an immune reaction is taking place in a patient. Such a reaction may be directed against cellular antigen on his own cells, for example as part of the pathogenesis of autoimmune disorders or against tumor antigens on neoplastic cells, or directed against donor-specific antigens in case of organ transplantation. Immunological investigations based upon living tissue cells as antigen material have been used very much within the field of cancer research during the last decade. In the majority of experiments a few long-term established cell lines have been used as source of antigen in investigations of different patients. Thus, the test has often been performed across a histocompatibility barrier, where the cultured tumor cells and the effector lymphocytes in cellular immune reactions are carrying different tissue type antigens. In a personal series of investigations of the immune reaction in human transitional cell bladder carcinoma, one long-term established cell line from a transitional cell bladder carcinoma, HU 456, was used to measure the lymphocyte-mediated cytotoxicity against bladder cancer cells in a cytotoxicity test originally described by Takasugi and Klein, illustrated in Fig. 24.1. As control of the specificity of the reaction, two other established cell lines were used as target cells in parallel experiments, a cell line from normal urothelium, HU 609, and an osteosarcoma cell line, SAOS-2. By comparing

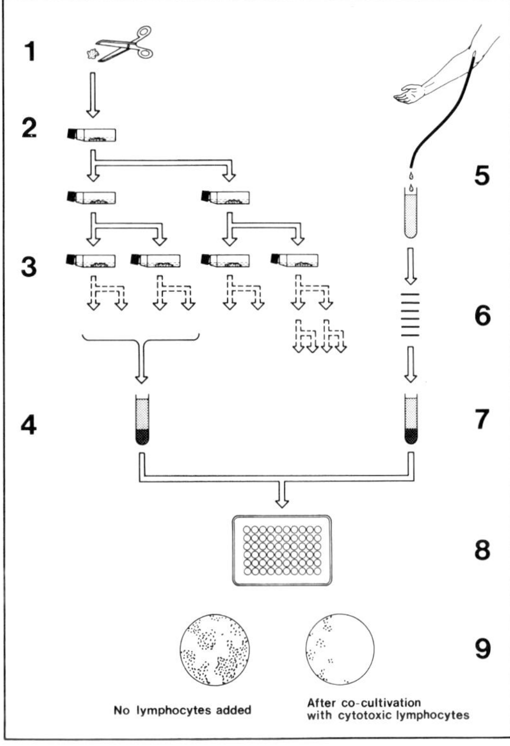



Fig. 24.1. *Lymphocyte cytotoxicity test*
1. The tissue is minced into small pieces, and added in suspension to culture bottles. 2. Primary mono-layer tissue culture of the cells. 3. Multiple subcultivations leading to an increase in cell number available. 4. Cells in monocellular suspension. 5. About 50 ml of peripheral blood is collected. 6. Fractionation of the leucocytes. 7. Pure lymphocytes. 8. Tumor cells and lymphocytes are co-cultivated in 20 µl wells in a microtissue culture tray. 9. Magnification of the bottom area in the micro-wells after 44 hours of co-cultivation of target cells and effector lymphocytes. The lymphocytes have been washed off, and the target cells are fixed and stained for optical counting.
The reduction of the number of surviving cells in wells with lymphocytes added, compared with the cell number in wells without lymphocytes, represents the lymphocytemediated cytotoxicity.

the reactivity of lymphocytes from a group of bladder cancer patients to the reactivity of lymphocytes from control patients, we were able to demonstrate a tumor type specific cytotoxic immune reaction on the background of a non-specific cytotoxicity.

The non-specific cytotoxicity was, however, very strong, and the value of the cytotoxicity test in clinical oncology remains rather limited. This evaluation of the cytotoxicity test is in accordance with the results obtained in several other centers, and it may even include other tests for cellular immune reaction against tumor-associated antigens.

Theoretically it may be assumed, that much better results can be obtained from tumor im-munological investigations, if it is possible to use freshly prepared autologous cell material as antigen. Thus, long-term established (months to years) cell lines may have lost tumor-specific antigens, or an immune reaction may be directed towards individually specific antigens not present on an allogenic cell line. Or an immune reaction against common tumor type specific antigens may even be blocked by a histocompatibility difference between target cells and effector cells. It can also be necessary to investigate cellular material from a tumor at different stages of the malignant disease, as the antigenicity may change with time, and this particular phenomenon may even be essential for the further existence of the tumor in the organism.

The possibility of repeated biopsies by means of

Table 24.1. *Estimation of quantity and nature of antigen material required in various immune techniques*
A: The material from a fine needle biopsy of a solid mass lesion is sufficient.
B: The material from a fine needle biopsy of a solid mass lesion is insufficient.
Humoral techniques: detection of antibody in serum or plasma.
Cellular techniques: detection of specifically sensitized lymphocytes

| | Nature of antigen | | | Amount |
| *Immune techniques:* | Whole cells | | Solubi-lized | of antigen |
| | Alive | Dead | | |
|---|---|---|---|---|
| *Humoral:* | | | | |
| Single radial immunodiffusion | − | (+)* | + | B* |
| Immunoelectrophoresis | − | (+)* | + | B* |
| Immunofluorescence | + | + | − | A |
| Immunoenzymatic histochemestry | + | + | − | A |
| Haemagglutination inhibition | − | − | + | B |
| Complement fixation | + | + | + | B |
| Complement dependent cytotoxicity | + | − | − | B |
| Antibody dependent cell-mediated cytotoxicity | + | − | − | B |
| | | | | |
| *Cellular:* | | | | |
| Cytotoxicity, visual counting | + | − | − | B |
| Cytotoxicity, radio labeled | + | − | − | B |
| Leucocyte migration inhibition | (+) | (+) | + | B |
| Leucocyte transformation | + | + | + | B |
| Leucocyte adherence inhibition | − | − | + | B |

* Immunodiffusion techniques are normally performed with soluble antigen. Methods have been described, however, using cellular material in the diffusion-gel, combined with chemical opening of the cell membrane.

ultrasonically guided fine needle aspiration is essential in this relation. This technique can be a convenient way to obtain freshly prepared autologous tissue with living cells for follow-up immune investigations of malignant diseases. However, when the aspiration is taken from a solid tumor, so few cells are obtained that it is insufficient for most immune techniques, unless the material can be augmented during a period of tissue culturing of the cells. In cases where the tumor creates effusions containing living malignant cells in suspension, for example ascites caused by ovarian carcinoma, or where there is a tumor cyst containing living malignant cells in suspension, it is often possible to obtain a sufficient number of cells for most immune techniques. But in these cases there is always contamination by other cell types such as leucocytes, macrophages, fibroblasts, or

Table 24.2. *Methods for preparative fractionation of mixed cell suspensions*

| 1:<br>Density gradient<br>centrifugation. | Much used within all kinds of cellular preparations, separates cells according to cell density. | As gradient can be used:<br>Percoll: forms continuous gradients spontaneously in an ultracentrifuge.<br>Sucrose.<br>Metrizamid.<br>Albumin. Ficoll. Ficoll-paque. |
|---|---|---|
| 2:<br>Unity gravity<br>sedimentation. | Much used within all kinds of cellular preparations. Cells are layered on top of the medium and sediments spontaneously, forming bands according to differences in size and density. | Fetal bovine serum, human AB + serum or Ficoll-70 can be used in most cases. |
| 3:<br>Aderence to<br>plastic or<br>glass surfaces. | Useful with tumor cells, that very often form adherent mono-layers in tissue culture medium supplemented with 10–20% serum on glass or plastic prepared for tissue culture. | Eagle's minimal essential medium (MEM), RPMI 1640 or Parker 199 may be used as culture medium supplemented with fetal bovine serum. Disposable tissue culture flasks. |
| 4:<br>Phagocytosis<br>dependent<br>separation. | Phagocytic cells may be removed by incubation at culture conditions with particulate iron followed by magnetic separation or density gradient separation. | Carbonyl iron. Culture medium. |
| 5:<br>Affinity<br>chromatography. | Much used in leucocyte separation, based on the existence of specific receptors on the cells. | Nylon or acryl wool columns. Specifically coated micro-beds or sepharose for cells with corresponding receptors. |
| 6:<br>Two-phase<br>partitioning. | Not much used, may be useful with cells with differences in surface charge. | Dextran – polyethylene – glycol. |
| 7:<br>Others. | Gel filtration, cell-electrophoresis, isoelectric focusing, cell sorting. | |

For further information se: N. Castimpolas (ed.): Methods for cell separation (*Plenum Publishing Corp.*).

non-malignant epithelial cells, and a fractionation of the cell suspension is necessary, before application of the cells in any test system. This situation is illustrated in Fig. 23.6.

A survey of the cellular material needed for various immune techniques is given in Table 24.1, in which can be seen whether the cell material from a fine needle biopsy of a solid mass lesion is sufficient, or augmentation of the material through a growth phase is needed. If, on the other hand, a large number of cells is available from malignant effusions or cystic cavities, fractionation procedures can be performed according to various principles as shown in Table 24.2.

Table 24.1 demonstrates, that the material, obtained by a fine needle aspiration of a solid mass lesion is sufficient only for immunohistochemical methods, immunofluorescence and immunoenzymatic techniques, and not for any of the tests for cellular immune reaction. The immunohistochemical techniques may be used to demonstrate antibodies in serum against cellular antigens, for example tumor-specific antigens. In most cases, however, it has not been possible to demonstrate tumor-directed antibodies in sera, neither when established cell lines were used in the investigations, nor when freshly prepared antigen material was used. The negative results frequently obtained when using fresh biopsy material may be due to coating of antigens by blocking factors, for example incomplete antibodies or antigen-antibody complexes. If this is true, it should be possible to eliminate this problem by means of a short tissue culture period, if necessary combined with trypsin treatment, at least 24 hours before harvesting the cells from the culture medium. Thus, even for the immunohistochemical methods, culturing of the cells may be necessary, and for the other immune techniques culturing of cells is needed to get a sufficient amount of material.

In a short series of experiments with fine needle aspiration biopsy material from solid mass lesions in human organs, we have been able to show that it is possible to obtain cell growth from this material by a simple culture technique, as shown in Fig. 24.2. Growth for 30 days or more was obtained in one of seven non-malignant cases, and seven of 18 malignant cases. Improved techniques are, however, necessary in order to have growth in all cases, and cytochemical methods for identification of the malignant cells are mandatory in order to exclude overgrowth by connective tissue cells.

Fig. 24.2. *Culture of fine needle aspirated cells*
1. The aspirated tissue in the needle is immediately (bedside) ejected aseptically onto the bottom of a dry 25 cm² disposable tissue culture flask. 2. Tissue culture medium is added, the flask is kept upside down. 3. The flask is kept upside down for 1.5–2 hours with a 5% carbon dioxide in air at 37 °C. 4. The flask is reverted to normal position, and the cell material is gently floated by the medium. The culture is now left untouched for 2–3 days before further handling.

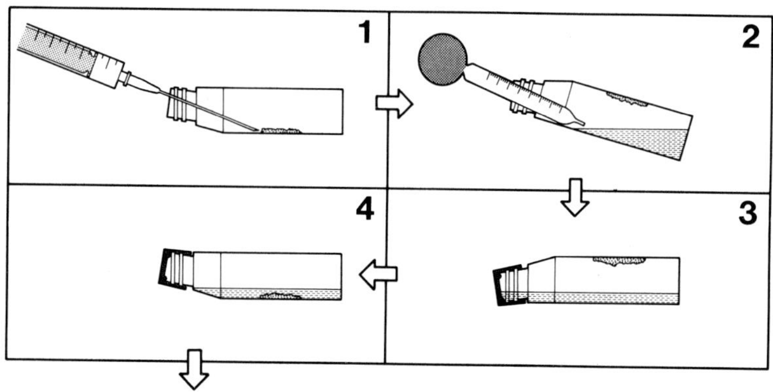

**Conventional cell culture technique**

# References


Baldwin, R. W. and Embleton, M. J.: Assessment of cell-mediated immunity to human tumor-associated antigens. *Int. Rev. Exp. Pathol.* 17:49, 1977.

Cerottini, J.-C. and Brunner, K. T.: Cell-mediated cytotoxicity, allograft rejection, and tumor immunity. *Adv. Immunol.* 18:67, 1974.

Doherty, P. C., Dietrich, G., Trinchieri, G. and Zinkernagel, R. M.: Models for recognition of virally modified cells by immune thymus-derived lymphocytes. *Immunogenet.* 3:517, 1976.

Gitling, D., Sasaki, T. and Vuopio, P.: Immunochemical quantitation of proteins in single cells. *Blood* 32:796, 1968.

Perlmann, P., Troye, M. and Pape, G.R.: Cell-mediated immune reactions to human tumors. *Cancer* 40:448, 1977.

Takasugi, M. and Klein, E.: A microassay for cell-mediated immunity. *Transplant.* 9:219, 1970.

Troye, M., Pape, G. R., Vilien, M. and Perlmann, P.: Characterisation of effector lymphocytes in allogeneic and autochtonous systems in patients with transitional cell carcinoma of the urinary bladder. In: Perspectives in Immunology, Ed. G. Riethmüller, P. Wernet, and G. Cudkewicz, *Academic Press,* New York 1978.

Vilien, M. and Wolf, H.: The specificity of the microcytotoxicity assay for cell-mediated immunity in human bladder cancer. *J. Urol.* 119:338, 1976.

Vilien, M., Holm, H. H., Gammelgaard, J., Larsen, S. and Hald, T.: Monolayer cultures of cells, originating from ultrasonically guided fine needle aspiration biopsies: to be published.

# CHAPTER XXV

# Alternative methods of biopsy

Edward H. Smith

Needle aspiration of lesions within the body have been carried out for many years, long before ultrasound was available. There are a variety of alternative approaches which include almost all the diagnostic modalities available today (Table 25.1).

## Physical examination

The simplest and most straightforward method consists of physical examination, especially palpation of a large mass with needle placement guided by the palpating fingers. Certainly in the situation where the mass is easily palpable this method would be acceptable. However, this is not commonly the case and even in these situations, one may be deceived as to the size of the mass by physical examination. In addition, biopsy of certain parts of the mass may be more likely to yield positive results than other areas (Figs. 25.1 and 25.2).

Table 25.1.

I. Palpation

II. Radiologic
    a. routine filming
    b. routine filming after contrast
    c. fluoroscopy
    d. angiography
    e. other

III. Computed tomography

IV. Ultrasound
    a. conventional B-scanning
    b. A-mode biopsy transducer
    c. B-scan biopsy transducer
    d. real-time

V. Other

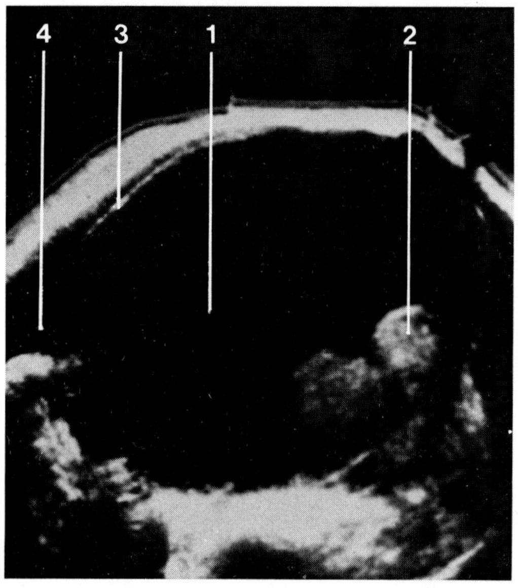

Fig. 25.1. *Malignant ascites*
Transverse scan of lower abdomen. 1. Ascitic fluid. 2. Tumor nodule. 3. Peritoneum. 4. Extravasated ascitic fluid after paracentesis.

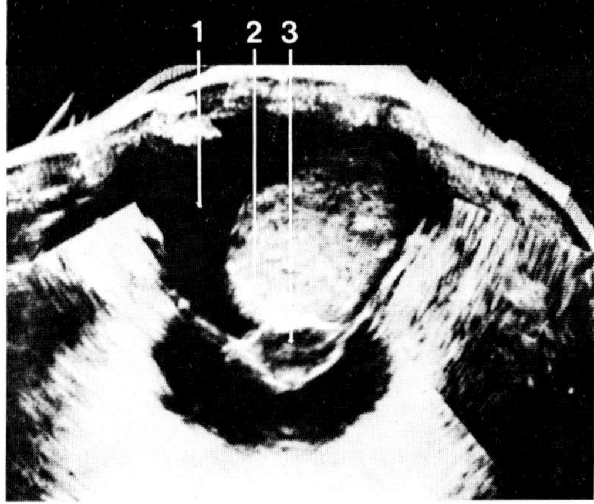

Fig. 25.2. *Malignant ascites*
Transverse scan of pelvis. 1. Ascitic fluid. 2. Metastasis to anterior surface of uterus from carcinoma of the breast. 3. Uterus. Ultrasonically guided biopsy revealed lesion to be metastasis rather than a new primary malignancy.

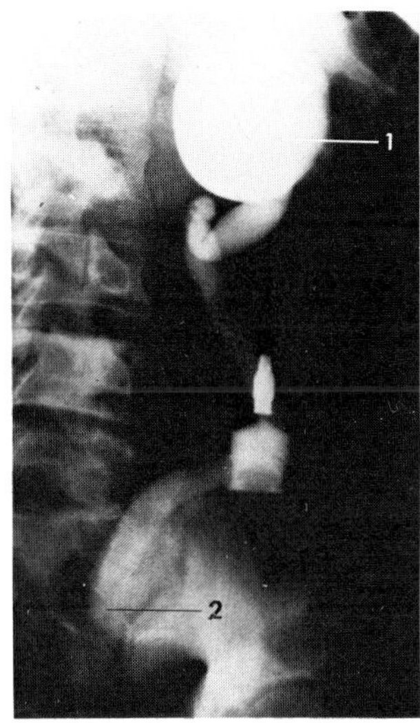

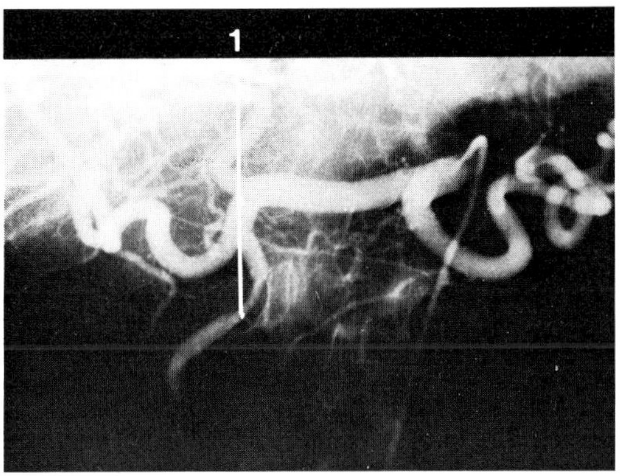

Fig. 25.5. *Carcinoma of pancreas*
Celiac angiogram 1. Encased gastroduodenal artery.

Fig. 25.3. *Hydronephrosis secondary to obstruction of the distal ureter by carcinoma of prostate*
Antegrade pyelogram. 1. Hydronephrotic renal pelvis. 2. Obstructed ureter.

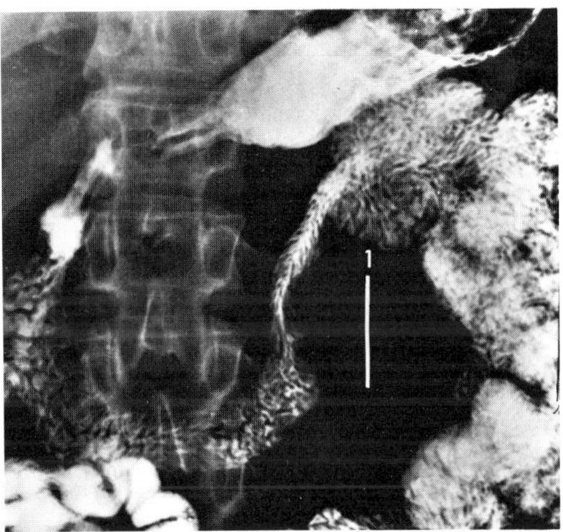

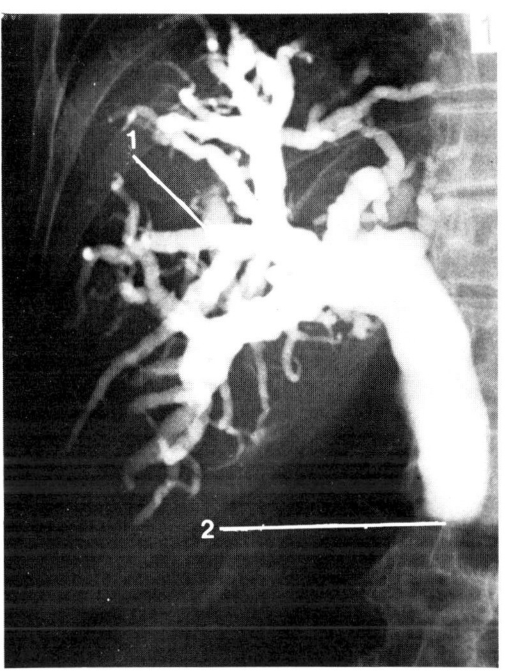

Fig. 25.4. *Lymphoma*
Upper gastrointestinal series. 1. Lymphomatous mass in root of mesentery.

Fig. 25.6. *Carcinoma of the pancreas*
Transhepatic cholangiogram. 1. Dilated biliary tree. 2. Obstructed common bile duct.

# Radiography

Another straightforward method consists of radiographic examination with identification of the mass on plain film. The needle can then be introduced, either in stages guided by further radiographs, or by a mark made on the skin with introduction of the needle and completion of the biopsy in one step. This method can be carried a step further by using contrast-enhanced radiographic methods to aid in the needle placement. The most common example of this would be in conjunction with excretory urography. Thus a mass or a hydronephrotic kidney may be identified on the urogram. With views in various projections, the center of the lesion can be identified and projected onto the skin. The approximate depth can be estimated, taking into consideration magnification, and needle puncture can then be carried out. In the case of a renal cyst, the puncture can be augmented by contrast injection into the cyst in order to more completely examine the cyst wall for nodules or asymmetrical thickening. If a hydronephrotic kidney is encountered, again contrast injection under radiographic or fluoroscopic guidance can be performed with opacification of the dilated collecting system to the point of obstruction, the so-called antegrade pyelogram (Fig. 25.3).

Obviously fluoroscopy can be performed, for example in association with a barium study of the gastrointestinal tract, with introduction of a needle guided by fluoroscopic visualization simultaneously of both the needle and the mass to be punctured (Fig. 25.4).

However, the barium study outlines only the contours of a mass and does not provide any information concerning its internal architecture. A somewhat more complicated procedure would consist of combining angiography with puncture guidance. Contrast material can be injected via a percutaneously placed vascular catheter with subsequent identification of either an area of tumor stain or tumor vasculature or encasement, the latter being the more common occurrence in pancreatic carcinoma (Fig. 25.5). Then, aided by hand injections of small amounts of contrast into the catheter, the vascular changes produced by the tumor can be visualized while fluoroscopically aiming the needle toward this area. If the appropriate equipment is available, one can fluoroscope simultaneously in two planes so that the depth of the lesion can be appreciated. Similarly percutaneous transhepatic cholangiography can be carried out with injection of radiopaque contrast material into the biliary tree. If an area of narrowing or irregularity can be detected fluoroscopically, then once again a needle can be advanced percutaneously toward the area under suspicion and aspiration biopsy carried out (Fig. 25.6).

Frequently lymphangiography reveals subtle changes in the paraortic abdominal lymph nodes which may or may not be enlarged. If a lesion is present elsewhere, i.e. in the chest, then it is often desirable to obtain tissue confirmation of the pre-

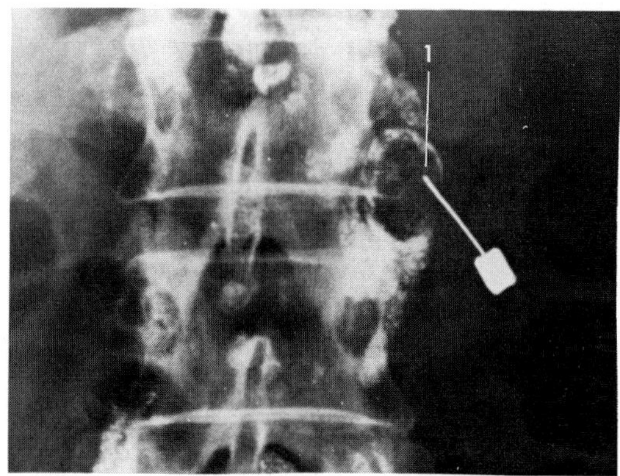

Fig. 25.7. *Lymph node biopsy*
Needle in lymph node metastasis. (Courtesy of Dr. Jack Wittenberg, Massachusetts General Hospital)

sence of involvement below the diaphragm so that the disease be correctly staged and appropriate therapy instituted. Therefore, after the lymphangiogram is performed and the suspicious lymph nodes identified, a biopsy needle may be placed percutaneously under fluoroscopic guidance. Again the availability of biplane fluoroscopy is an added advantage, especially for the biopsy of small lesions (Fig. 25.7).

## Radionuclide techniques

Radionuclide techniques may similarly be utilized to identify an area of abnormality with demarcation on the skin overlying the lesion and subsequent introduction of a biopsy needle. This can be done with either a static scan or in conjunction with a computer assisted dynamic flow study (Figs. 25.8 and 25.9).

The purpose of the latter is to determine the degree of vascularity of the lesion to be biopsied. Multiple projections of the lesion can be obtained so that the approximate depth of the lesion from the site of the biopsy can be obtained.

## A-mode ultrasound

Although not strictly an alternate method since it does make use of ultrasound, one can use the ultrasound A-mode scan to guide the introduction of the aspirating needle. This is particularly suitable for cystic structures where the needle tip can be visualized ultrasonically. As the fluid is aspirated,

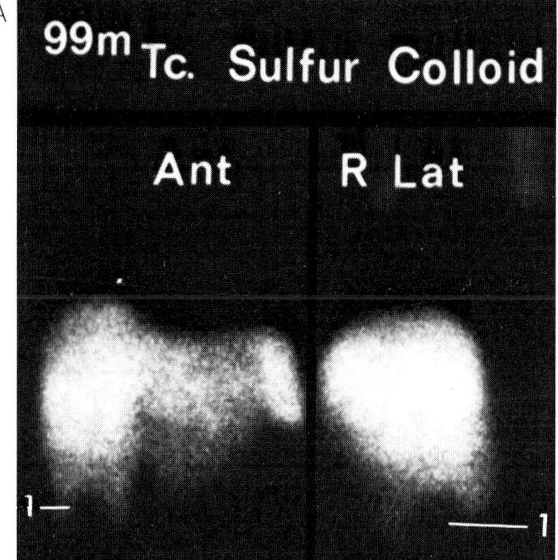


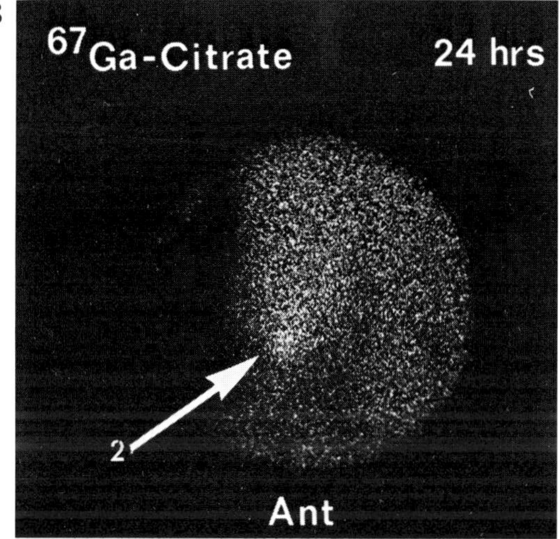


Fig. 25.8. *Liver abscess in patient with acute lymphocytic leukemia*
A. Perfusion scan. B. Gallium scan. 1. Focal defect tip right lobe of liver. 2. Increased uptake of gallium tip right lobe of liver.

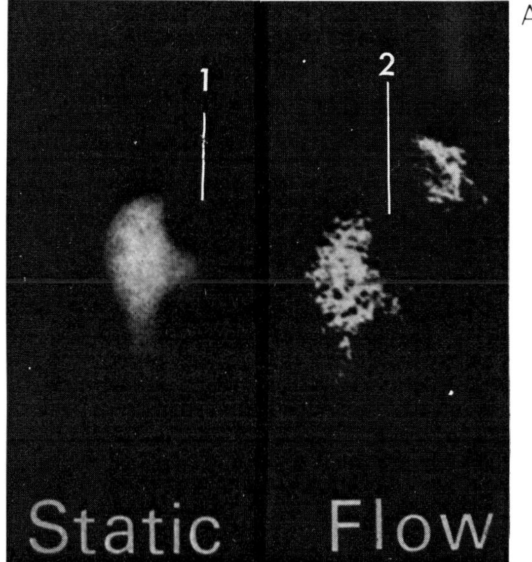


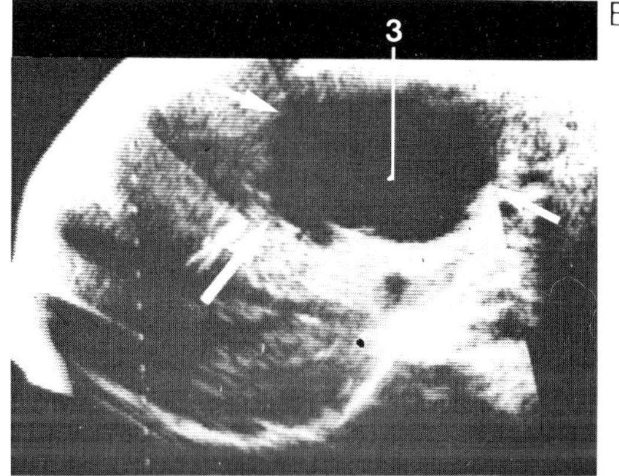


Fig. 25.9. *Liver cyst in patient with carcinoma of pancreas*
A. Static and dynamic flow nuclide scans. B. Transverse ultrasound scan through liver. 1. "Cold" area right lobe of liver on static scan. 2. Absence of flow to cold area on flow study. 3. Anechoic liver cyst (proven by aspiration).

the near and far wall of the lesion tend to approximate each other until finally they are superimposed and disappear when the lesion is emptied. An A-scan biopsy transducer with a central canal is available for this purpose.

## CT-scanning

Finally, the last method to be mentioned is that of needle placement under the direction of computed tomography. Using this technique, the lesion is localized on the CT scan, a point is marked on the skin overlying the lesion and a needle is then percutaneously introduced subcutaneously. The patient is then moved back into the scanner and the study repeated with either further introduction of the needle toward the lesion, or, if the needle appears to be off course, the needle is then removed or redirected. The process is repeated until the lesion is successfully negotiated. The advantage of this method is that the needle tip often can be identified and confirmed to be within the lesion

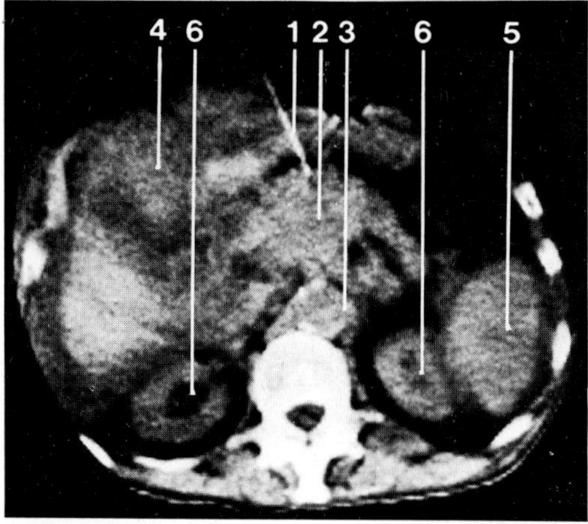

Fig. 25.10. *Computed tomographic guided biopsy of carcinoma of the pancreas*
Transverse computed tomogram through pancreas 1. Needle. 2. Pancreatic mass. 3. Aorta. 4. Liver. 5. Spleen. 6. Kidneys (Courtesy of Dr. Jack Wittenberg in *Radiology* 129:739–744, 1978).

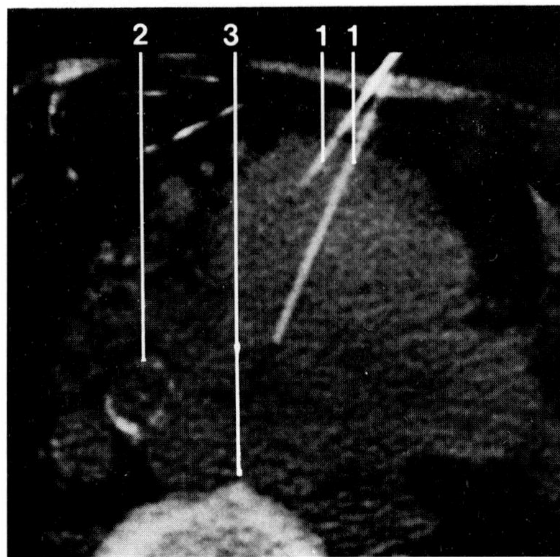

Fig. 25.11. *Computed tomographic guided biopsy of seminoma*
Transverse scan, detailed view. 1. Needles in mass (lymphadenopathy). 2. Calcified aorta. 3. Anterior edge of vertebral body (Courtesy of Dr. Jack Wittenberg, Massachusetts General Hospital).

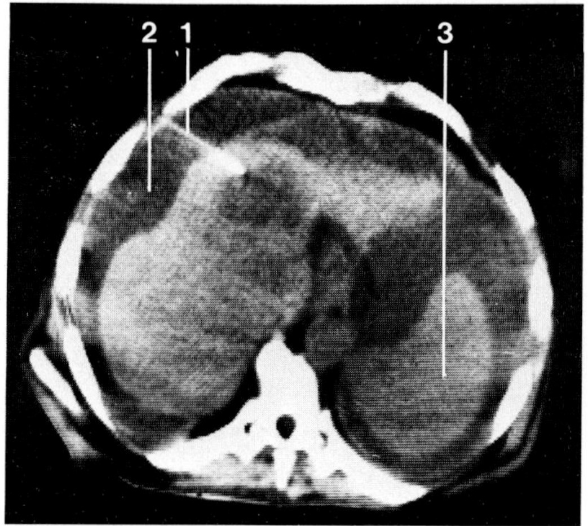

Fig. 25.12. *Computed tomographic guided biopsy of liver metastasis*
Transverse scan. 1. Needle in liver metastasis. 2. Ascites. 3. Spleen.

under question. Various systems have been devised to facilitate identification of the skin surface overlying a lesion under study. This method is most convenient when the needle pathway can be perpendicular to the skin surface. When the lesion is deep and the needle has to be severely angu-

lated, the procedure may be quite difficult and time consuming. In addition, it is not always possible to tell when the tip rather than the body of the needle is within the lesion (Figs. 25.10, 25.11 and 25.12).

All of the above methods can be utilized and are perfectly suitable in the appropriate situation. However, generally speaking, B-scan directed needle placement is the preferable method. Physical examination and radiographically guided needle placement including fluoroscopy do not allow two dimensional appreciation of the mass unless complex equipment is available.

In addition, the interior of the mass cannot be visualized so that the optimal site of biopsy within the mass cannot be determined. Angiography is a complex, invasive and time consuming method, but, on occasion, may be the only available approach if the lesion cannot be detected in any other way. For example, if the only evidence of a pancreatic mass is a localized area of tumor encasement of an artery or vein and this area cannot be visualized with ultrasound or any other modality, then obviously angiographically directed needle placement would be the method of choice. However, in most clinical situations, a mass is often associated with the tumor encasement. Obviously each clinical situation has to be considered individually, but, overall, ultrasound has proven to



Alternative methods

be the method having the widest application.

CT aided needle placement certainly is a possible method and frequently does allow identification of the needle tip within the lesion, certainly an advantage. However, it appears to be more time consuming, requiring the needle to be within the patient for extensive periods of time, compared to ultrasonically guided puncture and of course requires the availability of very expensive equipment. It would seem to make sense to use this type of needle placement guidance only in cases where the lesion can not be identified by ultrasound.

## References


Ferrucci, J. T. Jr. and Wittenberg, J.: CT biopsy of abdominal tumors: aids for lesion localization, *Radiol.* 129:739, 1978.

Haaga, J. R., Alfidi, R. J., Havrilla, T. R., Cooperman, A. M., Seidelmann, F. E., Reich, N. E., Weinstein, A. J. and Meaney, T. F.: CT detection and aspiration of abdominal abscesses. *Am. J. Roentgenol.* 128:465, 1977.

Jaques, P. F., Staab, E., Richey, W., Photopulos, G. and Swanton, M.: CT-assisted pelvic and abdominal aspiration biopsies in gynecological malignancy. *Radiol.* 128:651, 1978.

# Index